THE GINGER

& TURMERIC

COMPANION

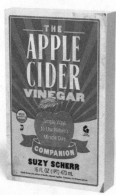
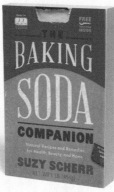
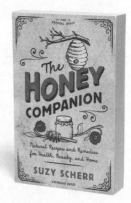

THE GINGER

& TURMERIC

COMPANION

Natural Recipes and Remedies
for Everyday Health

Suzy Scherr

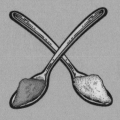

THE COUNTRYMAN PRESS
A division of W. W. Norton & Company
Independent Publishers Since 1923

This book is intended as a general information resource. It is not a substitute for professional advice and no recommendation in this book to eat, drink or use anything is intended to substitute for any prescribed medication. Consult your healthcare provider before changing your diet in any significant way and before eating any new foods or ingredients in significant quantities, especially if you are diabetic or suffer from any other health condition (and especially if you are taking any prescription drug), if you are pregnant or nursing, or if you have food or other allergies. Do the same before you offer any new foods, ingredients or products to children or use aerosol products around children.

Be sure to read the warnings that accompany some of the recipes about when not to eat certain foods, when not to use certain products, and when to seek immediate medical care instead of using any home remedy.

Any URLs displayed in this book link or refer to websites that existed as of press time. The publisher is not responsible for, and should not be deemed to endorse or recommend, any website other than its own or any content not created by it. The author, also, is not responsible for any third-party material.

For information about permission to reproduce selections from this book, write to Permissions, The Countryman Press, 500 Fifth Avenue, New York, NY 10110

For information about special discounts for bulk purchases, please contact W. W. Norton Special Sales at specialsales@wwnorton.com or 800-233-4830

Library of Congress Cataloging-in-Publication Data

Names: Scherr, Suzy, author.
Title: The ginger and turmeric companion : natural recipes and remedies for
  everyday health / Suzy Scherr.
Identifiers: LCCN 2019037334 | ISBN 9781682683767 (paperback) | ISBN
  9781682683774 (epub)
Subjects: LCSH: Ginger. | Cooking (Ginger) | Cooking (Turmeric) | LCGFT:
  Cookbooks.
Classification: LCC TX819.G53 S34 2019 | DDC 641.3/3832—dc23
LC record available at https://lccn.loc.gov/2019037334

Manufacturing by Versa Press

The Countryman Press
www.countrymanpress.com

A division of W. W. Norton & Company, Inc.
500 Fifth Avenue, New York, NY 10110
www.wwnorton.com

10 9 8 7 6 5 4 3 2 1

For my parents, the original dynamic duo

CONTENTS

HEALING TREATMENTS 108

BEAUTY SECRETS 154

AROUND THE HOME 198

INTRODUCTION

I bet I'm a lot like you. I want to be healthy and energetic, I want to feel good, and I want to *look* good—who doesn't? But, because I'm perpetually busy with work, family, and other assorted aspects of life, I can't (okay, fine, I *don't*) put a colossal amount of effort into achieving the ultimate wellness nirvana. I want to—really, I do—but the truth is, even though I know about spirulina and kombucha and bone broth and chia and goji berries and açai—I'm certain the science is there to back up the health claims around those foods—the ever-growing inventory of miracle products is overwhelming! I mean, just how many seeds, powders, roots, and greens can I actually cram into a smoothie before the day comes when my blender looks me in the eye and says, "Sorry, I just can't"?

The good news for all of us who want the best fuel for our busy lives and an easy ticket to health, beauty, and—what I believe is the real key to happiness—delicious food, is that there's an incredibly versatile and extremely powerful one-two punch that can get us there pronto. And likely, it's already hanging out in your spice cabinet. Ginger and turmeric, two mighty spices (cousins, actually) that have been used for thousands of years for both culinary and medicinal purposes, are not only easy but a pleasure to incorporate into your lifestyle. They will lead you squarely to vital, healthy, glowing territory, and you won't have to settle for "kinda healthy" or "healthy enough" anymore.

Ginger has been used in folk medicine, traditional Chinese medicine, and Ayurveda, to name but a few, and among its potent benefits are improved circulation, strengthened immunity, and defense against motion sickness. The oils in ginger are antiviral and contain antioxidants. Plus, ginger stimulates digestion and aids in transforming and transporting the fluids in the body, so it's super anti-inflammatory. It's also spicy and delicious.

Turmeric, a plant that's botanically related to ginger, packs an insanely healthful punch, too. It brightens skin, reduces inflammation, and even combats fatigue. It can improve digestion, support liver detoxification, boost circulation, and, because it's packed with antioxidants, including a compound called curcumin, it may even help fight off cancer-causing free radicals and Alzheimer's disease. Its gorgeous color lends itself to beautiful-looking food and also makes it a useful tool in tons of beauty applications.

I love both ginger and turmeric for their versatility in the kitchen—there's so much you can do with these spices! They enhance both sweet *and* savory dishes, so I use them all over the place: in teas, curries, soups, broths, chicken, cakes, even ice cream! From stir-fries to holiday cookies, these spark plugs can go all day. But in my house, we also turn to ginger and turmeric to solve all sorts of problems outside the kitchen: to treat a cold, soothe a headache, calm a cranky digestive system (or a cranky kid!), relieve skin irritations, and boost our overall immunity. I use them as part of my daily skin care and hair care regimen and have even been known to run to the spice cabinet when faced with a last-minute makeup emergency!

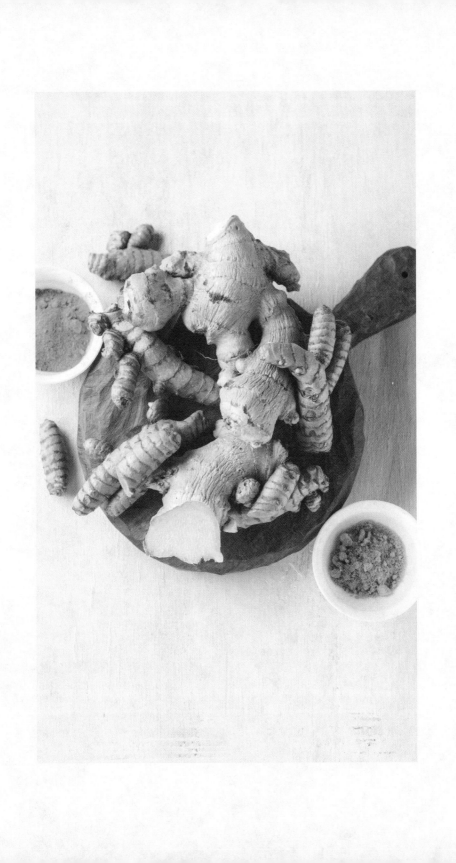

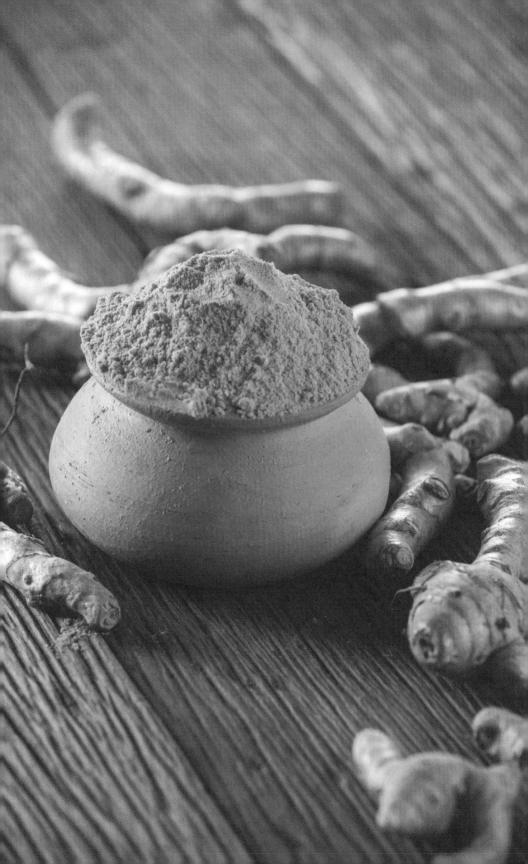

PART ONE

GETTING STARTED WITH GINGER AND TURMERIC

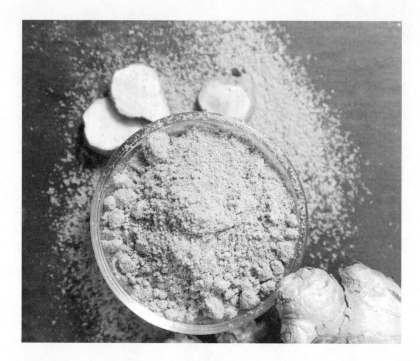

Meet Ginger

What Is It?

Ginger is the rhizome (more or less a root, but if you want to get super technical, it's actually an underground stem that grows horizontally, continuously producing roots and shoots to help the plant grow) of a flowering tropical plant known as *Zingiber officinale*. Originating in Southeast Asia, ginger has been coveted as a spice and a natural medicine since before history was even recorded. A long, long time. (Stifling a bad joke about deep roots!)

Culinary and Medicinal Uses in History

Because its history reaches so far back, it's hard to know exactly when ginger first came on the scene, but in all likelihood its origins date back about 5,000 years, to the tropical jungles of southern Asia. Historians' best guess is that the plant was first formally cultivated in India, followed shortly thereafter by cultivation in China.

About 3,000 years later, ginger made its way from India to the Middle East via trade routes and from there was sold to both the ancient Greeks and Romans, who prized it for its aroma, taste, and healing qualities. In fact, records show that ancient Rome taxed ginger when it came ashore at Alexandria. Around the time of the Spanish conquistadors, Europe began to discover ginger. That's when the practice of drying it began: to preserve its shelf life on the long voyages across the sea. By the 14th century, the wealthy in western Europe were bonkers for imported ginger, which was expensive (a pound was roughly the same price as a goat!). The only spice more popular was black pepper. In fact, Queen Elizabeth I is said to have been so fond of ginger that she created gingerbread men.

As western Europeans fanned out across the globe, ginger went with them. It eventually made its way to the warm, humid climate of the Caribbean, where it remains one of Jamaica's top exports. It is now grown in tropical countries around the world, with China and India still its largest exporters.

Health Benefits

There's good reason that spicy, pungent ginger has had such a long history in traditional and alternative medicine: it has all sorts of benefits for your body and brain. It is a powerful superfood: anti-inflammatory, antispasmodic, and packed full of a huge range of beneficial chemical compounds and nutrients, including vitamin C, magnesium, potassium, copper, and manganese. In large part, fresh ginger's superpowers—not to mention its amazing fragrance and flavor—come from the presence of gingerols, in particular [6]-gingerol, a chemical cousin of capsaicin (the compound that gives chilies their spiciness) and piperine (found in black pepper). When ginger is heated or dried, its gingerols are transformed into a different family of compounds called shogaols, which are also incredibly potent and, in some instances, even more beneficial for our health.

Much of ginger's street cred comes from its effectiveness as an anti-inflammatory agent, a nausea reliever, and a digestive aid. Modern research has found that the chemical compounds in both fresh and dried ginger are effective in easing stomach pain, aiding digestion, and relieving motion sickness as well as other types of nausea. Ginger is an age-old remedy for morning sickness during pregnancy, and studies have shown it to be a safe and effective way to help queasy mamas-to-be. In addition, ginger can help relieve nausea and vomiting after surgery and offers relief to patients undergoing chemotherapy.

When it comes to pain and inflammation, ginger is fierce! It has been shown to inhibit the production of pro-inflammatory cytokines and thus decreases the overall amount of inflammation in the body. And it's useful in easing postexercise muscle pain and joint pain due to inflammation from arthritis. Plus it gives over-the-counter pain medications a run for their money when it comes to relieving menstrual cramps.

But beyond its reputation as a nausea/digestion/anti-inflammatory triple threat, ginger has been shown to have a positive effect on blood sugar, blood pressure, and cholesterol. It can improve blood sugar levels and lower the risk of developing type 2 diabetes. And because of its high antioxidant content, ginger may help slow the aging process and might even fight off cancer cell growth. Plus ginger has antibacterial, antiviral, pain relieving, and fever-reducing properties, making it quite a force to be reckoned with when it comes to colds, respiratory infections, and the flu.

Ginger is generally considered safe and nutritious when included as part of a healthy diet. That said, don't go overboard with the stuff, because in this case too much of a good thing is pretty much a recipe for a handful of mild yet undesirable side effects, such as heartburn, gas, and diarrhea. So, eat it, but don't go nuts! And, as always, you should consult with your doctor before beginning any new health regimen, especially if you are undergoing chemotherapy, are taking blood thinners, or are pregnant. And always check with your pediatrician before using ginger to treat a child's illness or injury.

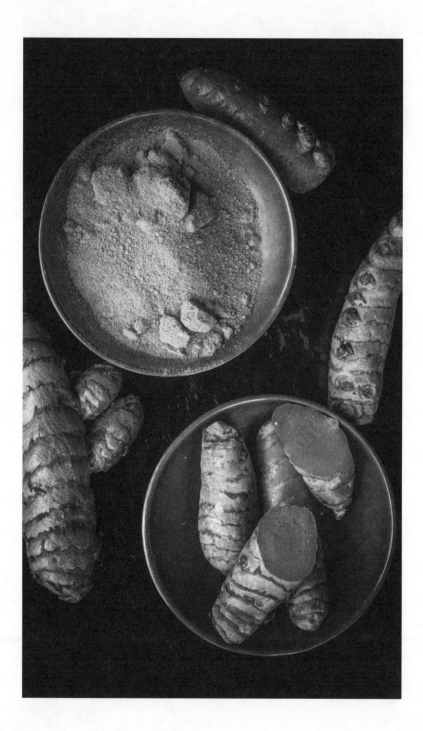

The Ginger & Turmeric Companion

Meet Turmeric

What Is It?

Turmeric, *Curcuma longa* in botanical speak, is a perennial flowering plant belonging to the ginger family that is native to Southeast Asia and the Indian subcontinent. Its beautiful yellow rhizome is the edible part of the plant and has been used for millennia as a dye, a ritual article, medicine, an antiseptic, and of course, a spice.

So, I bet you're wondering about the pronunciation, right? See, sometimes you go strolling along through life all la-di-da la-di-da without giving one single thought to how a word is pronounced. Like, say, turmeric. The word is tuRmeric. With two *r*'s. For whatever reason, it's easy to miss that first *r* after the *u* and pronounce it too-MARE-ic. It's actually TER-muh-ric, with the stress on the *first* syllable. (Though, to be honest, I don't really care how you pronounce it, just as long as you use it!)

Culinary and Medicinal Uses in History

Even though turmeric is trendy right now, it has been kind of a big deal for a pretty long time. Pick up any ancient Indian scripture, and you'll for sure come across tons of mentions of turmeric. It's known to have been in use since as early as 4000 BCE, playing a major role both as a culinary spice and in Ayurveda, the Indian system of holistic medicine also known as the "Science of Life." Some of its early applications are pretty fascinating, including the use of smoke from burning turmeric to relieve congestion. (Yep, they inhaled.) Early practitioners also used turmeric juice to heal wounds and bruises, and turmeric paste to treat burns and skin irritation, including smallpox and chicken pox. And its use was common in religious ceremonies and traditions (and still is in Buddhism, Hinduism, and throughout Southeast Asian society), where it was linked to fertility, luck, and the sun.

Turmeric reached China by 700 CE, East Africa by 800 CE, West Africa by the 1200s, and Jamaica in the 18th century. In 1280, Marco Polo stumbled upon it while on one of his legendary voyages to India via the silk route and was so struck by its similarities to saffron (a much more expensive spice), that he dubbed it "Indian saffron." From there, it was off and running on the culinary usage front.

Health Benefits

Science, Western medicine, and much of the rest of the world has started to wake up to what the East has known for a long time: turmeric is one of the world's healthiest foods. It contains several compounds with medicinal properties. Curcumin is the most active component of turmeric, making up between 2 and 6 percent of this spice. It's responsible for turmeric's distinctive color and flavor, and also is the element that gives it its anti-inflammatory, antibacterial, antitumor, brain-boosting, antioxidant superpowers.

When it comes to health, turmeric is definitely best known

for its anti-inflammatory properties, and quite a growing body of research supports the notion that this golden spice is a medicinal powerhouse. Inflammation is the body's natural way of protecting itself from infection, illness, or injury, and there are two types: acute and chronic. The redness, pain, heat, and swelling we associate with something like a sprained ankle or a sore throat is acute inflammation, and it occurs when your immune system calls in an infantry of white blood cells to surround and protect an area in distress. This kind of inflammation, while uncomfortable, is a sign that your body's systems are in good working order and doing what they're supposed to do. Sometimes, however, a body's immune system gets a bit glitchy and won't turn off. When this happens, you're looking at chronic inflammation, which can make an immune system go from healing damaged cells to harming healthy ones—sometimes even resulting in one of a variety of no-thank-you health concerns, including heart disease, diabetes, cancer, autoimmune diseases, and more. And the troubling part about chronic inflammation is that it can be silent: no pain, no swelling. No. Signs. While scientists are working to determine what exactly causes this kind of inflammation, one thing they know for sure is that lifestyle can play a pivotal role. Excess weight, stress, an imbalance in gut bacteria, and cigarette smoke have all been linked to increased inflammation. Doom and gloom, doom and gloom . . .

But wait—there's great news from Turmeric Town! Curcumin is incredibly anti-inflammatory. In fact, it's so powerful that, according to several clinical studies, it might be as effective as some anti-inflammatory drugs but completely natural. How? Well, I *could* totally impress you with some amazing molecular discourse because, *of course*, I know all about how turmeric inhibits the ubiquitous transcription factor NF-kB that binds DNA as a heterodimeric complex and causes inflammation, but I don't want to go too far over your head. (Ha ha ha. I'm kidding!) The truth is that the science around inflammation is pretty complicated. But know this: Curcumin fights inflammation at the molecular level. So, for the sake of our health, we should all be consuming more of it. That's not complicated.

What else can turmeric do for our health? What *can't* it do?! According to sources, including the National Institutes of Health, turmeric helps to fight oxidative damage and boost our body's own antioxidant enzymes. *Whuh?* Oxidative damage is one of the things that causes aging and many diseases. Laboratory studies also suggest that turmeric can improve brain function, fight Alzheimer's, reduce the risk of heart disease and cancer, and relieve arthritis. It's been shown to help with joint health, encourage healthy cholesterol levels, counteract the adverse effects of everyday stress on the body, support a healthy metabolism, and improve skin, mood, digestion, and blood sugar levels.

Sold? I thought so.

Unfortunately, I am forced to use a dirty word at this juncture. Patience. Uuuugh—I hate waiting! But the thing is, turmeric takes a bit of time to start working. Generally, people who start taking turmeric regularly will start seeing results after about three to four weeks. So, sorry to say, no instant gratification here, but the wait will be worth it, I promise.

Just remember, it's always a good idea to consult with your health-care provider before you start a new health regimen. Turmeric is generally safe for most people, but those with inflammation of the gallbladder or gallbladder stones, obstruction of bile passages, stomach ulcers, or diabetes should seek medical guidance before taking turmeric, especially in supplement form. As always, pregnant women should check with their doctor to be sure turmeric is a safe choice for them. And make sure to check with your pediatrician before using turmeric to treat a child's illness or injury.

Using, Buying, and Storing Ginger and Turmeric

Spicy, floral, and citrusy, the flavor and scent of ginger is unmistakable and inimitable. From gingerbread and ginger ale to stir-fries and soups, ginger is the must-have ingredient in so many delectable dishes. Turmeric's unique flavor, on the other hand, is sort of hard to describe. (Which is why you should just dive in headfirst and see for yourself!) Fresh or dried, it has a warm, bitter, peppery flavor and an earthy, mustard-like aroma. In a good way! Fresh turmeric has a slight sweetness to it, too. And when combined with other ingredients, both fresh and dried turmeric's culinary uses are pretty vast. It's a key ingredient in curry powder; adds depth, warmth, and color to all sorts of savory preparations;

and is also a fabulous complement to honey, making it a welcome addition to sweet dishes, too.

Once you start using ginger and turmeric, you'll surely find yourself adding them, both fresh and dried, to salads, grain dishes, eggs, marinades, soups, stews, and of course, tea. Oh boy, are you going to drink tea—this book has tea up the wazoo!

Knowing what to look for is the key to getting maximum flavor from both fresh and dried ginger and turmeric. Here's how to navigate the world of these two powerhouse ingredients.

Fresh Ginger and Turmeric

Fresh ginger and turmeric are both small and knobby-looking things, with smooth, firm flesh (creamy yellow in the case of ginger and bright, carrot orange in the case of turmeric) and a thin brown peel. Both fresh ginger and turmeric have a brighter, more in-your-face flavor than dried. They have thin skins that can be peeled prior to use, but I find that this is a matter of personal taste. I'm not bothered by the papery skin on ginger and turmeric and quite often leave it alone, but once you've worked with them for a while you'll figure out when it is and isn't necessary to scrape off the skin. To use fresh ginger and turmeric, you can slice it, julienne it, mince it, grate it on a Microplane or cheese grater, or juice it.

Look for fresh ginger and turmeric in the produce section where you shop. Ginger is pretty easy to find. It used to be that you could only get fresh turmeric at Indian or Asian markets and sometimes at specialty and health food stores, but I've noticed that my local supermarket behemoth has started to carry it, which is great news! Choose firm chunks of ginger and turmeric and avoid mushy, dried out, or wrinkly ones. Store the fresh rhizomes in the refrigerator in an unsealed plastic bag for a week or two. Or freeze it! I like to shred or grate it, press it into an ice cube tray, then stick it in the freezer. Once frozen, I pop the cubes out of the tray and store them in a freezer bag for easy use.

Dried Ginger and Turmeric

Dried ginger and turmeric, produced by peeling, boiling, drying (and then usually grinding) the rhizomes, can be found pretty much anywhere dried spices are sold. When ground, which is most often how it's sold, ginger is pale yellow in color, whereas turmeric is a vibrant, deeply orange powder that infuses recipes with bright, beautiful yellow-gold color. Both spices lose some of their pungency in the drying process, but dried ginger maintains a warm, spicy bite that is just a little bit sweet, and dried turmeric still has much of the same distinct earthy, woodsy, and floral flavor as fresh turmeric.

When choosing dried ginger or turmeric, one of the best ways to assess its quality is to give it a good sniff, as that's often a better indicator than anything else. If it smells like . . . well, if it doesn't smell much, it's old and/or poor quality, so take a pass. The ginger and turmeric you want to buy and use is aromatic and has scents of orange or lemon, pepper, and "spiciness." Because ginger and turmeric degrade in the presence of heat, oxygen, and sunlight, always store it in a cool, dry, and dark place. You know, like in your spice cabinet. (Duh.)

Substituting Dried Ginger and Turmeric for Fresh and Vice Versa

In many of the recipes in this book, you can successfully substitute dried ginger or turmeric for fresh, as well as the other way around, unless specifically noted otherwise. To do so, follow this general rule of thumb:

1 inch fresh rhizome = 1 tablespoon grated rhizome = 1 teaspoon ground (dried) spice

The Importance of Pairing Turmeric with Black Pepper and Healthy Fat

There is one vital tip when it comes to getting all the health benefits from turmeric: specifically, you have to consume it with black pepper. Curcumin all by itself is pretty difficult for the body to absorb, but a sort of chemical magic takes place when you pair it with black pepper that increases its bioavailability, making smaller doses more effective. So, don't forget to sprinkle some fresh pepper into any recipes that call for turmeric. And if you're taking a turmeric supplement, make sure to look for one that includes black pepper or its science-y name, piperine.

And, don't forget, turmeric is best absorbed if taken with some sort of fat, so take it with something like an egg, a handful of nuts, or—even better—check out the recipe for Golden Paste on page 53 for the easiest, tastiest delivery system of turmeric + fat.

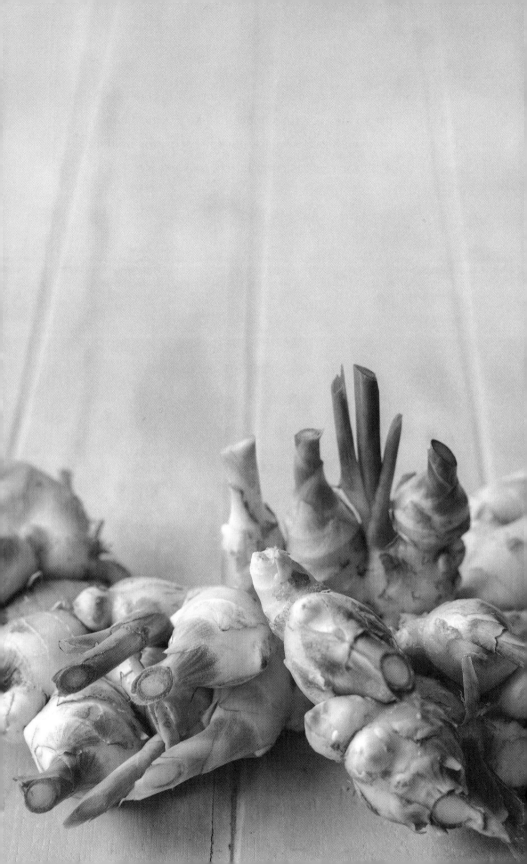

PART TWO

CLEVER WAYS TO USE GINGER AND TURMERIC AT HOME

DELICIOUS
RECIPES

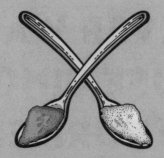

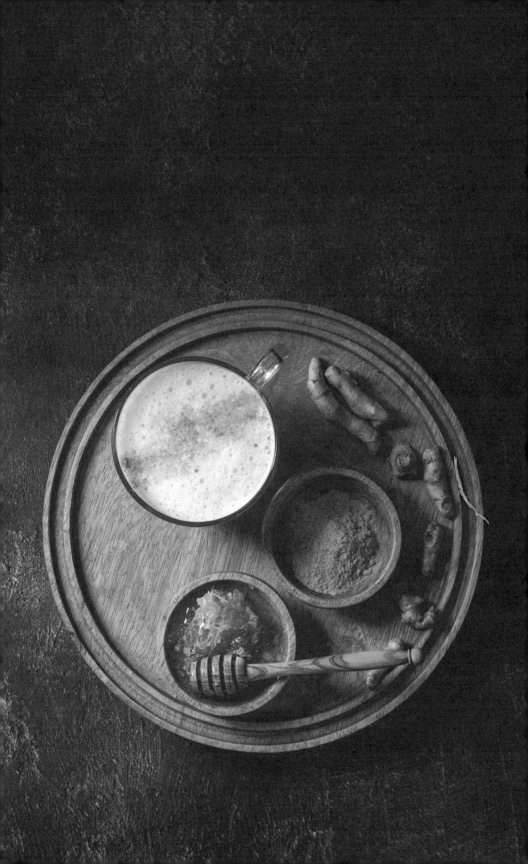

SIMPLE AND PERFECT
FRESH GINGER TEA ⓖ

I drink gallons of hot ginger tea, especially in the fall and winter, but really all year-round. I start just about every morning with some version of it. (Full transparency: after one single shot of espresso. I may kick that caffeine habit one of these days soon, and then it'll be fresh ginger tea out of the gates!) Most often, it's just a few slices of fresh ginger, a squeeze of lemon, and a shower of not-quite-boiling water. I steep it in a big mug or travel cup, which I sip from all day, adding more hot water as the tea disappears or gets cold. It's bracing and awakening but also soothing, which is why I think it does me right at any hour. Yes, it's anti-inflammatory, an amazing digestive aid, good for your heart, and even helpful in lowering cholesterol, but the real reason I drink it is because—you know what?—it's GOOD! I mean, it *tastes* good! Spicy and pungent and so easy to tweak to make it appeal to whatever mood I'm in, ginger tea is definitely a must-have around my house. Sometimes, I add a little honey or maple syrup if I need sweetness. Often, I add black pepper and turmeric and occasionally even a shake or two of ground cinnamon for added flavor and health benefits. But most of the time, straight-up ginger tea is just the thing. This recipe makes a very generous mug of tea. Some might say it serves two, but, as discussed, I like to drink a lot of it. This is how I roll.

Serves 1 or 2

One 2-inch piece fresh ginger, sliced thinly

2 cups water

2 tablespoons fresh lemon juice

1 to 2 sprigs mint (optional)

2 teaspoons honey, ideally raw, or to taste

1. Put the ginger and water in a pot and bring to a boil. Cover and let simmer for 20 minutes.

2. Once the ginger has been infused into the water, add the lemon juice and mint and allow it to steep for another 2 to 5 minutes.

3. Add the honey and, voilà, delicious.

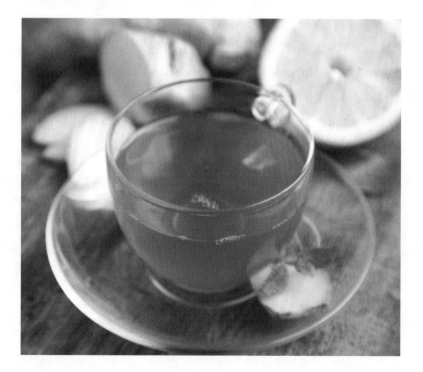

GOLDEN MILK (A.K.A. TURMERIC LATTE) G T

If you're looking for a super delicious beverage with health benefits that are through the roof, look no further. Golden milk—a creamy, warm beverage—is, hands down, one of the easiest ways to get more turmeric into your diet. But, judging from the fact that every hipster coffee and juice joint now seems to have some sort of tricked-out, cashew-dusted, hemp milk–steeped, holiday-scented version of golden milk on the menu for $7, it is apparently also one of coolest ways to get more turmeric into your body, too. A riff on the traditional Indian *haldi doodh*, which is typically just half a cup of hot milk mixed with a tablespoon of ground turmeric, this version kicks things up a bit. Calling for a little healthy fat in the form of coconut milk as well as a pinch of black pepper (both of which help your body absorb turmeric's nutrients) plus a touch of sweetener and warming spices, this drink will keep you healthy and so "on trend."

Serves 1

½ cup coconut milk

1 tablespoon raw sugar, 1 tablespoon pure maple syrup, or 2 teaspoons raw honey

4 teaspoons grated fresh turmeric, or 1 teaspoon ground

1 teaspoon grated fresh ginger, or ¼ teaspoon ground

⅛ teaspoon ground cloves or nutmeg

A few grinds of black pepper

Pinch of kosher salt

¾ cup water

1. Whisk together all the ingredients in a small saucepan and bring to a boil.

2. Remove from the heat and let the mixture steep for 5 minutes. Pour into a mug—if using fresh turmeric and ginger, strain the mixture, using a fine-mesh sieve—and serve.

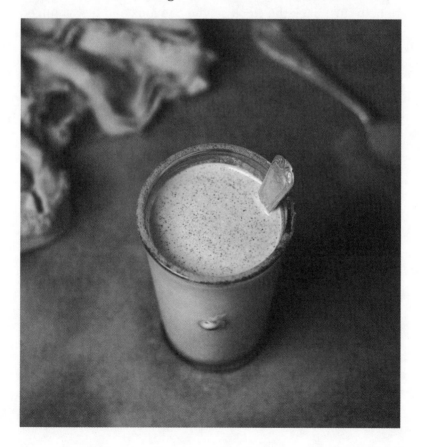

ANTIAGING TEA G T

You know what they say: "The best defense is a good offense."
Wait—is that what they say? Maybe it's "The best offense is
a good defense." Either way, when it comes to fighting the
signs of aging, there are no truer words. But the thing is, the
most powerful antiaging treatments don't come in sleek little
tubes of lotion or bottles of skin serum. Nope, true antiaging starts on the inside. In this powerful and delicious elixir,
turmeric and white tea touch rings like the Wonder Twins
to help turn back the clock so you can look and feel younger.
Both turmeric and white tea contain sky-high levels of antioxidants, which protect your skin's integrity by preventing
free radicals from destroying its texture and elasticity. Plus,
turmeric, with its anti-inflammatory superpowers, can help
calm such conditions as arthritis, eczema, and inflammatory
bowel disease and can help your body adapt to stressors,
such as environmental toxins and lack of sleep. All of which
is to say that I think there's a pretty good chance the Fountain
of Youth is flowing with *this* stuff.

Serves 1

1 cup water

1 teaspoon ground turmeric, or 1 tablespoon grated fresh

2 teaspoons loose white tea leaves or 1 tea bag

¼ teaspoon ground black pepper

¼ teaspoon ground ginger

1 teaspoon raw honey, or more to taste (optional)

1. Heat the water in a small saucepan until very hot but not boiling. Add the turmeric and white tea and allow to steep for 5 minutes.

2. Add the pepper, ginger, and honey, if using, stirring well to incorporate all the ingredients. Pour into a mug—if using loose tea or grated turmeric, strain the mixture, using a fine-mesh sieve—and enjoy your tea in small sips, gently shaking or stirring if the liquids and solids separate.

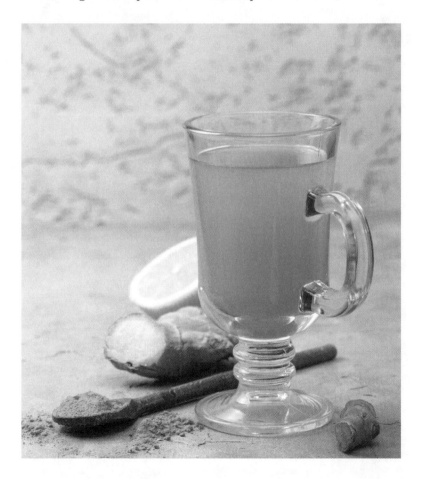

ANTI-INFLAMMATORY PINEAPPLE, WATERMELON, AND TURMERIC SMOOTHIE (T)

Whether you suffer from digestive issues or allergies, have just seriously rocked it at the gym, are recovering from surgery, or have some other kind of persistent inflammation, meet your new best friend. This light, refreshing, sweet, and tangy

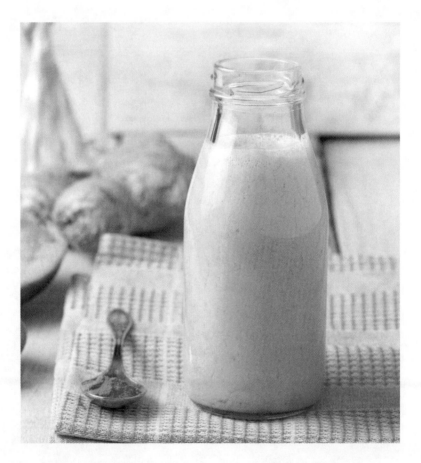

smoothie may taste like a trip to the tropics but is actually a powerful way to help your body take things down a notch (or five)! With fresh watermelon, pineapple, mango, coconut water, and turmeric (all of which bring mad anti-inflammatory skills to the table), let's just say this cool and frosty sipper tastes a whole lot better than anything you'd find in your medicine cabinet! Using frozen fruit instead of ice ensures a smoothie that's, well, smooth and not watered down in the least. And for refreshment in a flash, prep a bunch of freezer bags with ready-to-go, preportioned watermelon, pineapple, mango, and turmeric. That way, when you want to make this smoothie, all you have to do is dump the contents of one of your freezer bags into the blender, add the coconut water, and blitz away!

Serves 1

1 cup coconut water

4 cups cubed frozen watermelon

2 cups cubed frozen pineapple

2 cups cubed frozen mango

1 teaspoon ground turmeric, or 1 tablespoon peeled and grated fresh

Combine all the ingredients in a blender and blend until smooth. Drink immediately.

HOMEMADE GINGER BEER (AND MY FAVORITE GINGER MARGARITA) G

First thing's first: Let's get the ginger *ale* vs. ginger *beer* distinction out of the way. *What's the difference?* you wonder. Ginger beer is fermented with yeast to create carbonation (yes, the fermentation does result in a teensy amount of alcohol, though typically less than 1 percent, like kombucha or vanilla extract), whereas ginger ale gets its fizz from being force-carbonated with carbon dioxide. Also, ginger beer has real actual ginger in it, so it's full of spicy, pungent ginger flavor, whereas ginger ale is usually much sweeter, with very little (if any) real ginger in it. From a flavor perspective (and, honestly, from a health benefit standpoint), there's really no comparison. Ginger beer knocks the pants off ginger ale. My favorite part of this recipe, aside from its delicious result, is that you can make it in about an hour, and it'll be ready the next day for simply sipping over ice or mixing into cocktails like Moscow Mules, Dark and Stormys, or—my fave—ginger margaritas. And don't let the idea of having to track down champagne yeast turn you off. It's incredibly easy to find, any homebrew supply store will stock it—or perhaps you've heard of this new thing called the Internet? It's over there, too.

Makes about 2 quarts ginger beer

8 ounces fresh ginger, peeled and minced

2 quarts water

¾ cup packed dark brown sugar

¾ cup fresh lime juice

¼ teaspoon champagne yeast

1. Mix together the sugar, ginger, and 1 quart of the water in a saucepan. Bring to a boil, stirring to dissolve the sugar. Remove from the heat, cover, and let steep for 1 hour.

Continued

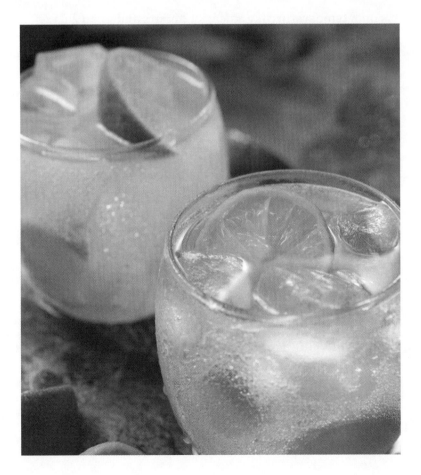

2. Strain the syrup through a mesh strainer and then use a funnel to pour the strained liquid into an empty 2-liter soda bottle.

3. Add the lime juice and remaining quart of water to the bottle until the liquid level is 2 to 3 inches from the top (you may not need to use all the water). Sprinkle the yeast on top of the liquid in the bottle.

4. Gently squeeze the bottle until the liquid comes to the neck, then screw the cap on tightly. Let the bottle sit at room temperature for at least 12 hours and up to 2 days, or until the bottle feels firm when squeezed. (Don't let the mixture ferment too long at room temperature! The pressure will continue to build and you could end up with a geyser or even an exploded bottle on your hands.)

5. Once the bottle is firm, store your ginger beer in the refrigerator and drink it within a week. Now, hurry up and make My Favorite Ginger Margarita!

My Favorite Ginger Margarita

This is the margarita you've been waiting for! Make it with your very own homemade ginger beer, fresh lime juice, and reasonably good-quality tequila (preferably 100 percent agave, but let's start at nothing in a plastic jug with a handle, mmk?). It's as if a margarita and a Moscow Mule had a baby. A miracle of life. If you like things spicy, do what I do: garnish your drink with a couple slices of fresh jalapeño to kick up the heat.

Serves 1

2 lime wedges

Coarse salt, for rimming glass (optional, but is it really?)

2 ounces tequila

2 tablespoons fresh lime juice

½ cup ginger beer

2 to 3 teaspoons simple syrup, to taste

1. To prepare the glass: Run one of the lime wedges around the rim and press it into a small plate of coarse salt. Fill the glass with ice.

2. Pour the tequila, lime juice, ginger beer, and simple syrup directly into the prepared glass. Stir well and garnish with a lime wedge.

Note: To make simple syrup, combine 1 cup of water with 1 cup of sugar in a small saucepan. Bring it to a simmer, stirring, to dissolve the sugar, then remove from the heat, let cool, and store in the refrigerator until ready to use. It'll keep pretty much indefinitely.

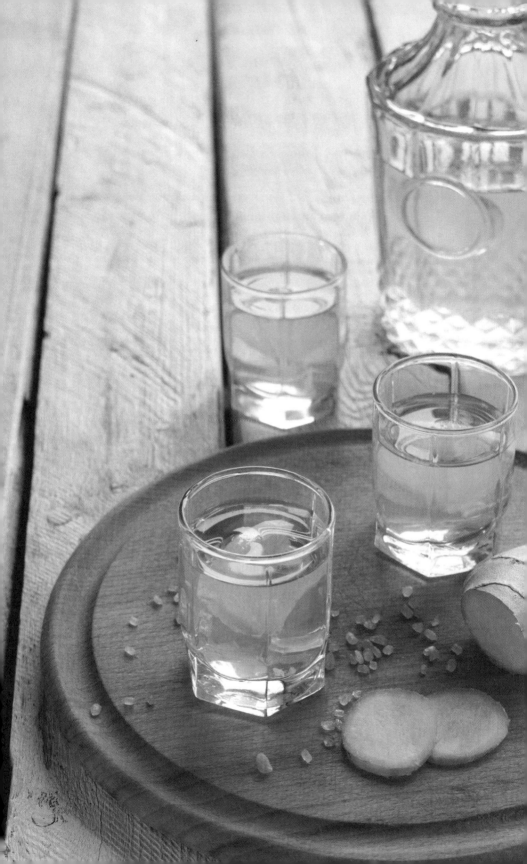

DIY GINGER LIQUEUR Ⓖ

This crazy simple recipe for homemade ginger liqueur, infused with tons of zingy fresh ginger, orange zest, and vanilla, is one of my favorite ways to fool, *ahem*, delight family and friends. In case you didn't know, if you put delicious things into some kind of liquor and let it steep for a good while in a cool, dark place, you wind up with liqueur that tastes like that delicious thing you put in it. It's one of those tricks that will make you look like an alchemist or an artisan or both when really all you did was shove some stuff in a bottle and wait around for something to happen. Perfect for gift giving, this delicious, complex, and truly elegant liqueur will perk up a cup of tea or hot cider, add a bright and festive touch to a simple glass of sparkling wine, and lend a boozy-sweet kick to cocktails of all sorts. You can tweak the recipe a bit to suit your tastes and/or the season. For example, swapping out the brandy for vodka and/or subbing in lemon or even grapefruit zest for the orange gives the finished product more of a sunny, summery finish. Adding some whole spice, such as star anise, cloves, or a cinnamon stick, to your brew gives you a final result that is perfectly suited to all those warm, fall- or winter-spiced beverages that just scream "holiday season"! But no matter how you tweak it, this indispensable and incomparably delicious liqueur will surely become a fixture of your home bar.

Makes about 4 cups liqueur

Continued

6 ounces fresh ginger, peeled and thinly sliced

1 whole vanilla bean, split lengthwise

2 cups sugar, or 1 cup honey

1 tablespoon loose leaf chamomile tea (optional)

2 cups water

Zest of 1 orange

2 cups brandy

1. Combine the ginger, vanilla, sugar, chamomile tea (if using), and water in a small saucepan and bring to a boil. Lower the heat and simmer for 20 minutes. Remove from the heat and let the syrup cool.

2. Without straining it, pour the cooled syrup into a glass jar or container with a tight-fitting lid. Add the orange zest and brandy. Seal and shake the jar, then let steep for 1 day.

3. The next day, remove the vanilla bean and let the mixture steep for 1 day more.

4. Strain the liquid through a few layers of cheesecloth or a coffee filter while funneling into a clean glass bottle or jar. Cap (or cork) and let the mixture mellow for 1 more day.

5. Store the liqueur at room temperature for up to a year.

WHITE MISO, TURMERIC, AND GINGER DRESSING G T

It's common knowledge that, when it comes to salad, it's not the vegetables or even the crunchy add-ins that make or break the finished product—it's the dressing! Fortunately, this dressing is incredibly easy to make—it takes less than five minutes! All you need are a few simple ingredients, a jar, and the ability to shake your fist (and, by all means, your groove thang, if you think it'll help). Here, turmeric, mellow white miso, ginger, and a few other flavorful friends come together in a gorgeous, vibrant dressing that you'll love drizzled on salad—but don't be surprised if you find that you can't stop there. This stuff is great on grain bowls, drizzled over seared fish, tossed with cold noodles, and even stirred into hummus. Fresh turmeric will give you the best flavor and health benefits, but ground, dried turmeric works, too.

Makes about 1 cup dressing

⅓ cup unseasoned rice vinegar

¼ cup mirin

¼ cup neutral-flavored oil, such as grapeseed or canola

2 tablespoons finely grated carrot

2 tablespoons white miso

1 tablespoon peeled and finely grated fresh ginger

2 teaspoons peeled and finely grated fresh turmeric, or
　½ teaspoon ground

1 teaspoon toasted sesame oil

Whisk together all the ingredients in a small bowl. Cover and chill. The dressing can be stored in the refrigerator for up to 1 week.

GINGER BROTH Ⓖ

Aside from bone broth, which is having some kind of a moment right now, broth is sort of a misunderstood food, often overlooked by home cooks, regarded as boring, difficult to make, unnecessary, and/or easily replaced with something from a can. So, let me set the record straight: homemade broth is *important*, it's easy to make (you chuck stuff in a pot and walk away), and it's so much more delicious than anything you'll find on a grocery store shelf. Knowing how to make a tried-and-true broth is foundational to knowing how to cook good food, which is why (along with stock, which is similar to broth though not quite the same) it is among the first things we learn how to make in culinary school. If you've got a good broth or stock, then you're well on your way to a good sauce or soup or wherever you're headed with your cooking. If your broth is too bland, salty, or otherwise subpar, you're not likely to end up with something that tastes very good. Simple as that. Chicken and/or beef broth is tasty and widely useful in the kitchen, but this light, bright, ginger-infused broth is equally indispensable and brings the added benefit of being really good for you: immunity-boosting, anti-inflammatory, and comforting yet energizing. You'll want to sip this stuff as is; however, it is even better to use it to make heartier soups with the addition of such yummy add-ins as rice noodles, chicken and/or mushrooms, or whatever combination of soup ingredients you like. Use it in place of water when cooking grains or as the poaching liquid for fish. And if you don't have time to watch over a simmering pot, toss all the ingredients for the broth into a slow cooker, set it to low, and let it go for eight hours.

Makes about 8 cups broth

8 cups water

1 medium yellow onion, peeled and quartered

2 celery stalks, cut in to 2- to 3-inch pieces

One 2-inch knob fresh ginger, peeled and cut into
    ½-inch pieces

6 large garlic cloves, peeled and roughly chopped

2 teaspoons whole black peppercorns

2 tablespoons fresh lemon juice

3 sprigs thyme

Salt

1. Combine all the ingredients in a large stockpot, adding salt to taste. Bring to a boil, then lower the heat to a simmer and cook for about 1 hour.

2. Strain the liquid through a fine-mesh sieve and discard the vegetables. Allow the broth to cool, then store in jars or other airtight containers with tightly fitting lids in the refrigerator for up to a week or in the freezer for up to 3 months.

CHILE, LIME, AND GINGER SALT Ⓖ

Flavored salts (or finishing salts, as they're sometimes called) are the secret weapon behind many a mouthwatering meal. Simply salts that've been infused with natural ingredients, such as herbs, spices, and fruits, they add a final pop of flavor and crunch to food. This lime and ginger salt is all at once spicy, earthy, tangy, and bright, making it work as a take-it-over-the-edge flavor enhancer for all manner of dishes, from grilled, sautéed, or fried foods to fresh salads, simple sliced tomatoes, eggs, and even plain yogurt drizzled with honey. It's also fairly mind-blowing sprinkled over vanilla ice cream. Just saying . . . And it makes a great gift: fill a cute little tin or jar, add a pretty ribbon, and you're officially a food gifter. Just remember, a little goes a long way with this stuff; all you need is a pinch sprinkled over a finished dish for a delicious result.

Makes about 1 cup salt

½ cup grated lime zest (from about 6 limes)

½ teaspoon crushed red pepper flakes

3 teaspoons ground ginger

1 cup coarse, flaky salt (I like Maldon salt, but you could use sel gris, coarse sea salt, or even kosher salt)

Spread the lime zest on a sheet of parchment or waxed paper; let dry overnight. Combine the dried zest, red pepper flakes, ground ginger, and salt in a medium bowl. Stir with a fork to break up any chunks. Store in an airtight container in a cool, dry place for up to 3 months.

ESSENTIAL TURMERIC AND BLACK PEPPER PASTE (A.K.A. GOLDEN PASTE) T

Think of this recipe as a sort of all-purpose turmeric short-cut that you can use to make tons of other dishes in minutes. It's the turmeric equivalent of cake mix, bouillon cubes, or frozen juice concentrate, except without 4,000 preservatives and artificial who-knows-what. And *so* good for you. Not that it's difficult to add a spoonful of turmeric to whatever you're cooking, but as we know, taking turmeric in combination with black pepper and some sort of fat is the most surefire way to get that precious curcumin into the ol' machine. Here you have all the key players premixed and ready to rock, so all you have to do is add a dollop to your next stir-fry, smoothie, tea, nut butter, soup, stew, or curry. In fact, you'll probably find that once you start making this stuff, you won't be able to stop dreaming up new ways of using it, which is why you might even consider making a double batch: one for now and one for the freezer. Fill ice cube trays with the paste, then freeze them, and you'll have preportioned little flavor bombs on hand for your obsessive recipe tinkering.

Makes about 1⅓ cups

½ cup ground turmeric

½ cup water

⅓ cup extra virgin coconut oil, olive oil, or flaxseed oil

2 to 3 teaspoons freshly ground black pepper

1 teaspoon ground cinnamon (optional)

1 teaspoon ground ginger (optional)

1. Combine the turmeric and water in a small saucepan and bring to a boil over high heat. Lower the heat and simmer for about 10 minutes, or until the mixture is reduced to a thick paste. If necessary, add more water, a tablespoon at a time, to keep the consistency thick, like paste.

2. Remove from the heat and allow it to cool to room temperature or just slightly warmer, then stir in the oil, pepper, cinnamon, and ginger (if using). Transfer to a glass or plastic container with a tight-fitting lid.

3. Store the paste in the refrigerator for up to a month or in the freezer for up to a year.

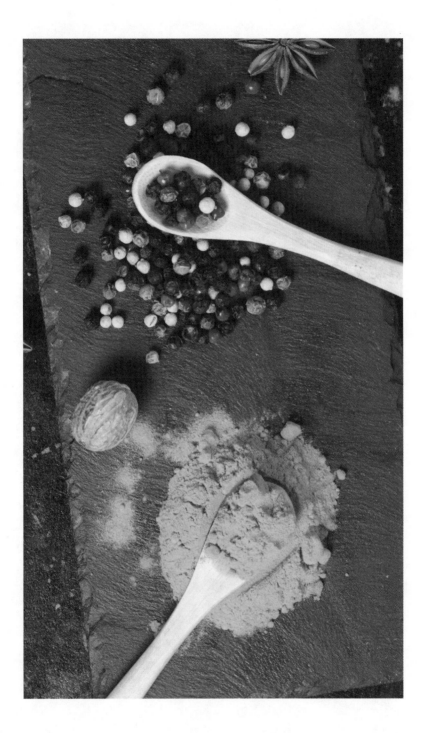

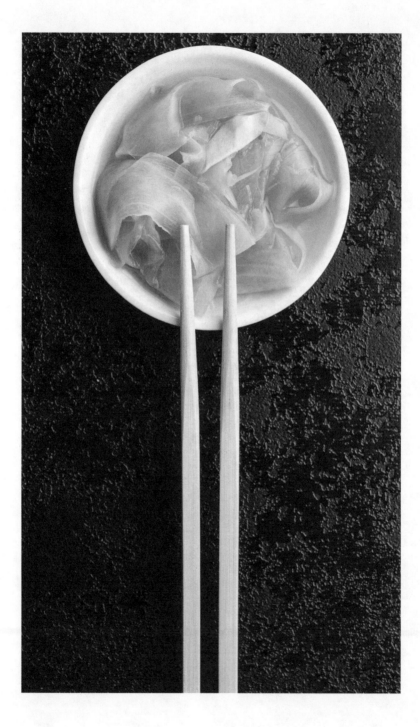

The Ginger & Turmeric Companion

PICKLED GINGER, SUSHI STYLE ⓖ

Many sushi devotees would argue that the *gari* (pickled ginger) that comes alongside any sushi order is the most important part of the plate, because its job is to cleanse your palate between bites of *maki* and *nigiri* and whatnot. I seriously love sushi and could eat it every day, but in all honesty, I have always been pretty lukewarm on that little pink pile. To me, it's always a bit too sweet, and I have to confess to being a little weirded out by the color. It turns out gari is *supposed* to be pink, but only because it's *supposed* to be made with young ginger, which is naturally pink. Most of the stuff you'll find at a run-of-the-mill sushi joint is not made with young ginger and, as such, is artificially colored. Because I am not content to simply dislike a food without putting up a fight—it's something I'm working on, I swear—I had to tinker a bit to find a version of pickled ginger that I actually *want* to eat. This super easy recipe turns out an all-natural, snappy, spicy, just-sweet-enough pickle that is not only great with sushi but adds something special to salads, sandwiches, and rice bowls, too. Be sure to use unseasoned rice vinegar here; the seasoned kind contains added sugar and salt.

Makes about 1 cup pickled ginger

Continued

1 large piece ginger (about 4 ounces), peeled

1 medium radish (optional, for use by those who absolutely *must* have their ginger tinted pink)

1 teaspoon kosher salt

¼ cup unseasoned rice vinegar

¼ cup water

¼ cup sugar

1. Using a vegetable peeler or mandoline, slice the ginger and radish, if using, into paper-thin strips. Transfer the ginger to a bowl and sprinkle with the salt. Set radish aside. Stir ginger and salt until well combined, then set aside for 30 minutes.

2. Using your hands, squeeze any excess liquid from the ginger, then transfer to a clean, heatproof glass jar or container with a tight-fitting lid. Add the radish.

3. Combine the rice vinegar, water, and sugar in a small saucepan and place over medium-high heat, stirring until the sugar dissolves. Bring the mixture to a boil, then immediately pour the vinegar mixture over the ginger and radish, if using. Allow the jar to cool, uncovered, to room temperature, then seal and place in the refrigerator for at least 24 hours before diving in.

4. The pickled ginger will keep in the refrigerator for at least a couple of months.

QUICK AND COMFORTING BUTTERNUT SQUASH AND TURMERIC SOUP ⓣ

There are two kinds of people in this world: soup people and non-soup people. Soup people (my husband and younger daughter) are the people who eat soup year-round, no matter the weather, no matter the meal; they love soup and will eat it anytime, anywhere. Non-soup people (me and my elder daughter) may like soup just fine, but they are most likely to eat it in the cooler months, when it feels like "soup weather." (I could break down the sociology even further into subcultures that include broth-based-soup eaters and chilled-soup eaters, but I'll save that for *The Soup Companion* . . .) This recipe is for soup people and non-soup people alike, perfect for warming everyone up from the inside out. Vibrantly colored, aromatic with the flavors of the cooler seasons, and scented with turmeric's signature peppery earthiness, this soup is in heavy rotation in our kitchen from around Halloween to "Hey, I just saw a daffodil." I love it because it's super quick and weeknight friendly, incredibly nourishing, and easily adapted to incorporate whatever winter squash you like and/or happen to have on hand (pumpkin, acorn squash, even sweet potato, which isn't a squash, but it works). My husband loves it because, well, because he's a soup person; my kids love it because it's neon

Continued

orange, and orange food is exciting for some reason. I make the recipe in batches large enough to feed a small village and freeze it to enjoy through the fall and into the winter (after which I'm *done* with soup; bring on the salads instead!). Whatever kind of soup eater you are, you'll be happy to have this one in your rotation.

Serves 4 to 6

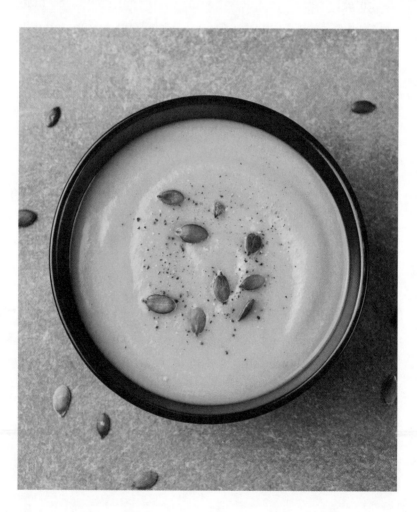

2 tablespoons extra virgin olive oil

1 small white onion, cut into small dice

2 garlic cloves, minced

One 2-inch piece fresh turmeric, peeled and thinly sliced, or
2¼ teaspoons ground

¼ teaspoon ground cinnamon

1 teaspoon sea salt

Freshly ground black pepper

1 large butternut squash (about 3 pounds), peeled, seeded, and
cut into 1-inch chunks

6 cups stock (any kind)

Optional garnishes: toasted seeds (use the seeds *inside* the
squash!), chopped toasted nuts, crumbled goat cheese,
sliced pears, beans, fresh herbs, plain yogurt, coconut milk

1. Heat the olive oil in a large saucepan or Dutch oven over
   medium heat. Add the onion and cook, covered, stirring
   occasionally until tender, 6 to 8 minutes. Add the garlic,
   turmeric, cinnamon, salt, and pepper to taste and cook for
   about 30 seconds more, or until aromatic.

2. Add the squash and stock and bring the mixture to a boil.
   Lower the heat to a simmer and cook for about 20 minutes,
   or until the butternut squash is fork tender.

3. Using an immersion blender (or standard blender, working
   in batches), puree the soup. Serve unadorned or sprinkled
   or swirled with your desired garnishes.

GINGER- AND COCONUT- MASHED SWEET POTATOES Ⓖ

The idea of a sweet potato mash has honestly never done much for me. I have a funny relationship with sweet potatoes in the first place in that I always enjoy them when I eat them, and I buy them often, but for some reason I usually have to really psych myself up to cook them. I suspect I'm not alone in this. I think it may have something to do with the fact that they're kind of sweet but not actually all *that* sweet—an indecisive food. How am I supposed to commit to a food that seemingly won't commit itself to a category? *Show yourself, tuber! Are you sweet or aren't you?!* Although I take a firm stance that a little butter and salt is all you need to make most foods delicious, when it comes to sweet potatoes, I need more. This recipe is more. With bright ginger and luxurious coconut milk, it is decadent, perhaps even holiday worthy (with nary a marshmallow in sight), yet quick and easy enough to whip up any night of the week. And, yes, it happens to be vegan, Paleo, gluten-free, and incredibly good for you, with fiber and healthy fat and tons of antioxidant power. There are lots of varieties of sweet potatoes, not all of them orange; make this mash with any kind you like.

Serves 4 to 6

Continued

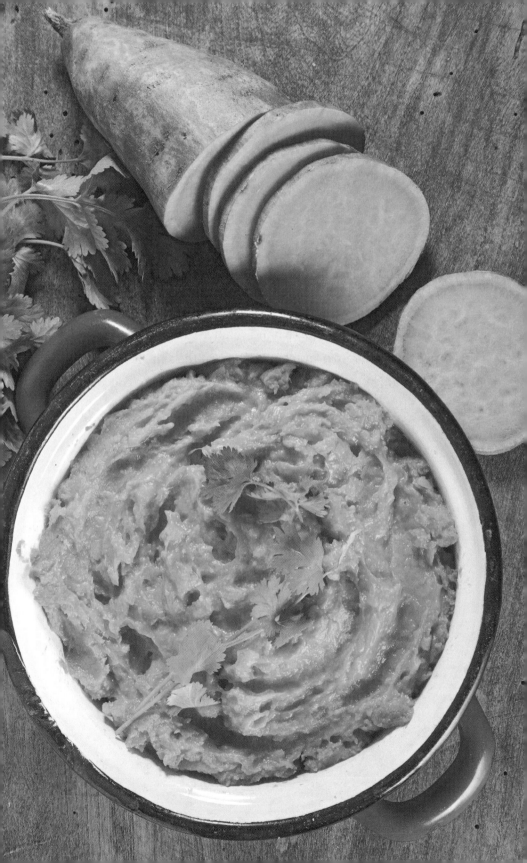

4 large sweet potatoes

½ cup unsweetened coconut milk

1 tablespoon peeled and grated fresh ginger

¼ teaspoon kosher salt

Freshly ground black pepper

Ground cinnamon (optional)

1. Preheat the oven to 400°F. Pierce the sweet potatoes several times with a sharp knife and bake on a foil-lined baking sheet for 45 minutes to 1 hour, until tender.

2. When cool enough to handle, halve the potatoes and scoop the flesh into a large bowl. Discard the skin. Mash thoroughly with a potato masher or ricer. Add the coconut milk, ginger, salt, and pepper and cinnamon (if using) to taste, and mix well to combine.

3. If you're not serving the potatoes right away, allow them to cool, then refrigerate for up to 3 days. You can rewarm the potatoes in a microwave on HIGH in 30-second intervals, stirring each time, until hot, or place them in a bowl over a pot of simmering water, stirring occasionally.

HONEY-ROASTED
WHOLE CARROTS Ⓣ

I'm going to make a bold claim right now. Ready? This recipe is going to change the way you think about carrots. Or, at the very least, how you think about cooked carrots. Forget steaming, forget boiling, forget slicing. Forget mushy and limp. These carrots are deeply flavored, earthy with turmeric and whole cumin, just slightly chewy at the edges, and melt-in-your-mouth amazeballs. Although you could easily serve them as a side dish to elevate something like roast chicken or, frankly, just about any other entrée, you could also toss these gems onto, say, a bed of greens. Top that with some chopped nuts, plain yogurt, or tahini; a handful of fresh herbs and pomegranate seeds; and a drizzle of good extra virgin olive oil, and then, well, then you'd have yourself one heck of a main course salad. If you happen to have fresh turmeric on hand, use it here—the flavor and texture will be ever-so-slightly superior to using dried, though you can't go wrong either way.

Serves 4

1 pound carrots, ideally on the thinnish side, scrubbed, greens removed (halve very large carrots lengthwise)

3 tablespoons olive oil

1 tablespoon finely grated fresh turmeric, or ½ teaspoon ground

Continued

2 teaspoons whole cumin seeds

2 teaspoons whole coriander seeds

½ teaspoon crushed red pepper flakes

Kosher salt

Freshly ground black pepper

1 tablespoon fresh lemon juice

1. Preheat the oven to 450°F.

2. Toss the carrots with the olive oil, turmeric, cumin, coriander seeds, and red pepper flakes on a parchment-lined baking sheet and season liberally with salt and black pepper. Roast, shaking the pan occasionally, until the carrots are evenly browned and tender (but not totally soft), 20 to 25 minutes.

3. Remove from the oven and drizzle with the lemon juice. Serve.

Note: I almost never peel carrots. If they're reasonably fresh, you really don't need to do so. Just give them a good scrub and get ready to roast. For the freshest carrots, grab a bunch at your farmers' market; or, at your local supermarket, look for carrots that are vibrant in color—the pigment fades over time, so the freshest carrots will pop with color.

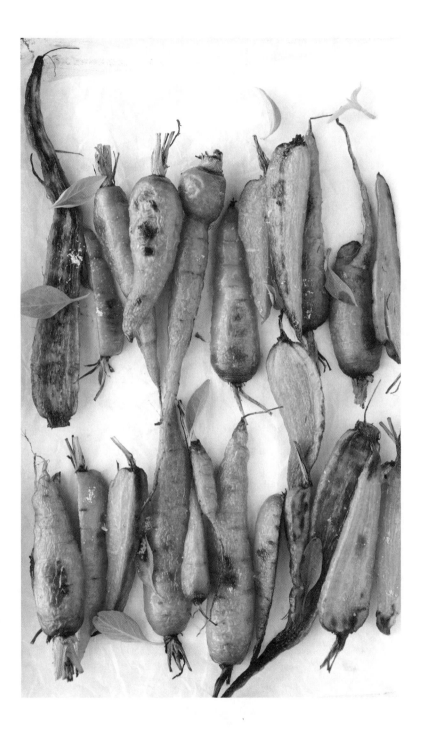

PERFECT YELLOW RICE G T

Yellow rice is exactly what it sounds like: rice that has been turned yellow (usually from turmeric). It's a delicious and simple accompaniment to all sorts of roasted and grilled meats and fish, a real crowd-pleaser that I've cooked many times for universally happy clients. Although I did have this one rather finicky "client"—who was five years old and lived in my house. In a desperate attempt to encourage my deeply rice-averse kid to expand her side dish horizons, I succumbed to buying a commercially produced package of yellow rice mix (full of sodium, artificial junk, and other additives that I don't usually feed my family), thinking that just maybe, if I found the rice equivalent of boxed mac and cheese (I *told* you I was desperate), I'd achieve some kind of breakthrough. And then, naturally, she loved it in all its processed glory. And, yes, I am aware that I brought that on myself. Thankfully, it turned out that the packaged stuff was simply a gateway to the real stuff, which is literally just as easy to make, even more delicious, and a great way to show off turmeric's gorgeous color. You can use virtually any kind of long-grain rice here, though if you're going with brown rice, you'll need to adjust the cooking time quite a bit.

Serves 4

1 cup uncooked basmati rice, rinsed

1 tablespoon unsalted butter, olive oil, or coconut oil

½ teaspoon ground turmeric

¼ teaspoon ground ginger

¼ teaspoon salt

⅛ teaspoon freshly ground black pepper

½ teaspoon onion powder

½ teaspoon garlic powder

2 cups chicken or vegetable stock

1. Combine all the ingredients in a medium pot.

2. Cover and bring to a boil; then lower the heat and simmer, covered, for 15 minutes.

3. Remove from the heat and let sit, still covered, for another 10 minutes before fluffing with a fork and serving.

SUSHI-ISH RICE BOWLS WITH CLASSIC GINGER-CARROT DRESSING Ⓖ

Rice bowls are big in our house. They make for a quick and easy weeknight meal and/or a satisfying desk lunch. They're extremely customizable, which is handy for managing assorted mealtime demands—*ahem*—requests from, say, small dining companions who may have some extremely specific ideas about what foods should and should not appear on their dinner plates and whether said foods should be allowed to touch one another. In other words, diners can pick and choose what ends up in their bowls. Burrito bowls, Indian rice bowls, Thai-style curry bowls, bits and bobs of whatever-is-hanging-around-the-fridge bowls—they've all come to my rescue on many a harried weeknight. But my favorite, hands down, and the bowl that ends up in my husband's lunch more often than not, is a sort of deconstructed sushi bowl. Fresh, bright fish and vegetables (or just vegetables) atop simple sushi rice are then adorned with toppings galore, including a homemade version of the ubiquitous sushi restaurant ginger-carrot dressing. Sushi bowl, poke bowl, Buddha bowl . . . whatever you want to call it, it's way better than calling it take-out!

Serves 4

2 cups sushi or short-grain rice (white or brown)

¾ pound *sushi-grade* raw fish, cut into bite-size pieces; leftover salmon (from recipe on page 76); or 1 pound cubed tofu, marinated in ¼ cup soy sauce, ¼ cup rice vinegar, and 1 teaspoon sesame oil

Ginger-Carrot Dressing (recipe follows)

SOME TOPPINGS TO CONSIDER:

1 or 2 avocados, peeled, pitted, and sliced

1 bunch scallions (white and light green parts), thinly sliced

2 seedless cucumbers, sliced

1 cup shelled edamame

Furikake (a dried seaweed, fish, and sesame seasoning, available at Asian markets)

Pickled ginger (for homemade see page 57)

Toasted sesame seeds

Crumbled nori sheets

Spicy mayo (mayonnaise plus sambal oelek)

Steamed spinach

Steamed sweet potato

Ponzu sauce

Pineapple

Peanut sauce

Sriracha

1. Prepare the sushi rice according to the package directions.

2. Divide the rice and fish or whatever protein you're using among bowls, then go bananas with the toppings. That's pretty much all there is to it!

Ginger-Carrot Dressing

Makes 2 cups dressing

½ cup vegetable oil

¼ cup rice vinegar

2 tablespoons soy sauce

1½ teaspoons sugar

1 teaspoon finely grated fresh ginger

1 medium carrot, peeled and roughly chopped

½ small yellow onion, roughly chopped

Kosher salt

Freshly ground black pepper

Combine the oil, vinegar, soy sauce, sugar, ginger, carrot, and onion in a food processor or high-speed blender and process until smooth; season to taste with salt and pepper. Store in an airtight container in the refrigerator for up to 2 weeks.

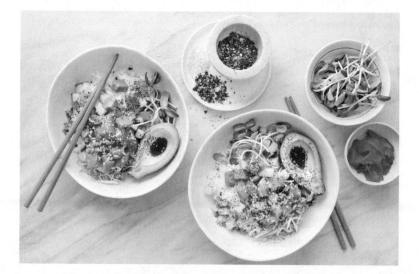

HALIBUT WITH
GOLDEN SAUCE Ⓣ

My mom gave me this recipe years ago. It is delicately flavored, absolutely beautiful to look at—as though it has been kissed by the sun—and one of my all-time favorite ways to use turmeric. And the best part, according to my mom, is that you can make any number of changes to it, including the type of fish, the citrus, and the herbs, and still end up with something that's both easy to prepare and worthy of company. Although she isn't a classically trained chef, she is one of the most inventive, spontaneous, problem-solving cooks (and people) I know. Just ask her about what she's served most recently to dinner guests and you'll see what I mean. The conversation could go like this:

MOM: I found out Jane and Tom lost power in the storm the other night, so I invited them over for dinner.

ME: That was nice of you. What did you make?

MOM: Well, it was last minute, so I made that chicken recipe, you know the one with the dried figs, almonds, and couscous?

ME: Yeah, that's a yummy one.

MOM: It is, although I was out of figs, so I threw in some dried apricots instead. Oh, and pistachios instead of almonds. I thought the color would be nice.

ME: Still sounds good.

MOM: It was! Oh, and it's a good thing I remembered that Jane is gluten-free; I served it over rice instead of couscous.

ME: I'm sure that worked.

Continued

MOM: Yeah, it did. I didn't have any chicken in the house, but it was fine—I real quick defrosted some fish and used that. And, after the fact, I realized I forgot the cinnamon.

ME: So, you made fish with apricots and pistachios.

MOM: Yeah, and I think I liked it better that way.

Serves 4

3 large lemons

1 tablespoon ground turmeric

½ teaspoon salt

2 tablespoons olive oil, plus more for cooking and serving

4 garlic cloves, minced

½ teaspoon saffron threads steeped in ⅓ cup hot water

1 bunch fresh cilantro or parsley, chopped

Four 6-ounce halibut fillets (or sea bass, cod, or really any fish you like)

Freshly ground black pepper

1 cup pitted green olives (optional)

1. Peel and remove the pith from two of the lemons, then thinly slice. Juice the remaining lemon. Place the lemon slices in a small bowl and toss with the turmeric, ¼ teaspoon of the salt, 2 teaspoons of the olive oil, and the lemon juice. Set aside.

2. Heat 1 tablespoon of the remaining olive oil over medium-low heat in a large sauté pan. Add the garlic and cook, stirring occasionally, for about 1 minute, or until it is fragrant

but not browned. Add half of the saffron infusion and simmer for another minute, until the liquid is reduced by about half.

3. Arrange the lemon slices on the bottom of the pan, reserving all the accumulated juices in their bowl. Scatter half of the cilantro over the lemon, then arrange the fish fillets in a single layer on the lemon slices. Sprinkle the fish with the remaining ¼ teaspoon of salt, pepper to taste, the remaining saffron infusion, the reserved juices from the lemons, the remaining cilantro, and the olives.

4. Increase the heat to medium-high, bring the liquid to a boil, lower the heat to low, cover, and simmer for 8 to 10 minutes, until the fish is just cooked through and flakes easily with a fork. Serve immediately, drizzled with remaining olive oil.

GINGER-SOY MARINATED SALMON ⓖ

I love salmon and am content to eat it prepared pretty much any way at all. Perhaps this is because it is such a versatile protein that works with just about any cooking technique. I like it grilled, broiled, steamed, pan seared, cured, smoked, raw, poached, roasted. I like it served hot. I like it served cold. (I will eat it with a fox. I will eat it in a box. I will eat it here and there. I will eat it anywhere!) One of my most favorite ways to cook salmon is as follows: simply marinating it in a salty-sweet, gingery bath, and then blasting it under the broiler just until it's caramelized on the outside and perfectly tender and silky within. The finished product is delicious served just from the oven, but it's also good at room temperature. Leftovers are really great on a salad or, need I remind you, in a rice bowl (flip back to page 70).

Serves 4

¼ cup white miso
¼ cup mirin
2 tablespoons unseasoned rice vinegar
3 tablespoons soy sauce
1½ tablespoons minced fresh ginger
2 teaspoons toasted sesame oil
2 tablespoons minced scallion
Four 6- to 8-ounce salmon fillets
Salt and freshly ground black pepper

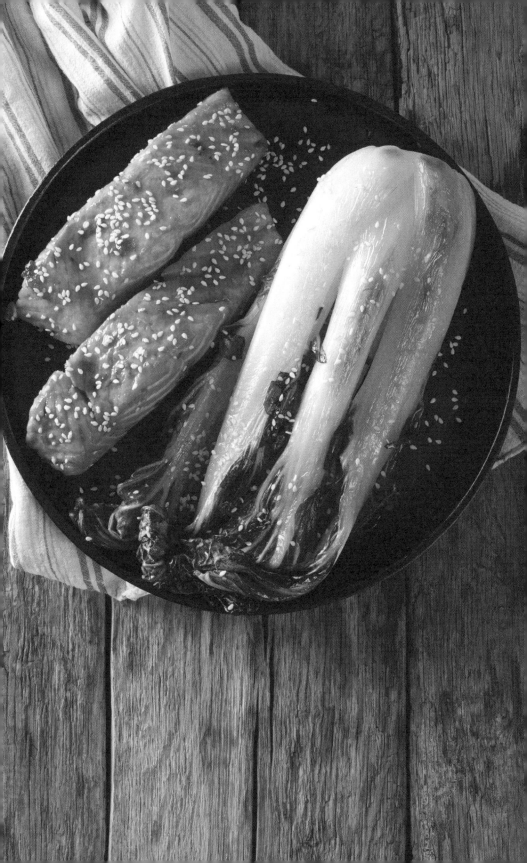

1. Combine the miso, mirin, vinegar, soy sauce, ginger, and sesame oil in a small bowl and whisk until smooth. Stir in the scallion.

2. Place the salmon fillets in a small baking dish, then pour the marinade over the fish. Turn the fillets a few times to coat them. Cover and let marinate in the fridge for 30 minutes, turning occasionally.

3. Remove the fillets from the marinade and season with salt and pepper. Discard the marinade.

4. Preheat your broiler. Place the fillets, skin side down, on a baking sheet or broiler pan. Broil them (without turning!) for 5 to 6 minutes, until the salmon is just barely cooked through and the top is beautifully caramelized. Serve immediately.

GINGER BBQ SHRIMP KEBABS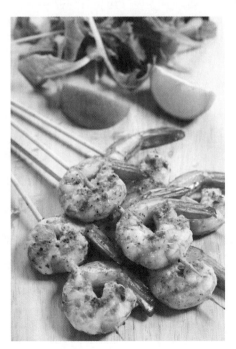

It's easy to fall into a cooking rut anytime, but come summer it's especially easy to fall into a grilling rut of burgers-dogs-chicken-repeat. Those foods, plus the occasional steak or vegetable kebab, are super tasty, so it's no wonder they get stuck on replay, but who wants to be bored? Life's too short for that. This summer, throw these sweet and gingery shrimp kebabs into the mix to liven things up. They're quick enough for a weeknight meal (and can even be made under the broiler or on a stovetop grill pan if it's not barbecue season), but are also the perfect one-handed food for entertaining—your guests won't even need to put down their drinks to eat them. Buy shelled and cleaned shrimp to save on prep time, thread them onto skewers, then toss 'em "on the barbie" with a quick shellac of gingery barbecue sauce (which, by the way, you'll want to use on all your other grilling standbys, too), and have dinner ready in no time.

Serves 4

SAUCE:

1½ cups apple cider vinegar

½ cup honey

½ cup ketchup

1½ tablespoons hot sauce

2 tablespoons minced garlic

2 tablespoons peeled and minced fresh ginger

1 teaspoon salt

SHRIMP:

2 tablespoons vegetable oil for grill

2 pounds jumbo or extra-large shrimp, shelled and deveined

½ teaspoon salt

1. Prepare the sauce: Combine all the sauce ingredients in a medium saucepan and bring to a boil over high heat. Lower the heat to medium-low and simmer, uncovered, stirring occasionally, for about 25 minutes, or until the sauce is thickened. Remove from the heat and set aside.

2. Prepare the shrimp: Soak eight to ten wooden skewers in water for 15 minutes. Heat a grill or grill pan to medium-high. Clean and lightly oil the hot grill.

3. Thread the shrimp on the prepared skewers. Grill until the shrimp begin to turn opaque, about 2 minutes. Brush them with the sauce, flip, and brush again. Grill until the shrimp are opaque throughout, about 3 minutes more. Serve with the reserved sauce.

CHICKEN TAGINE WITH OLIVES AND LEMONS G T

A tagine is a Moroccan stew. And it's also the name for the conical earthenware pot it's traditionally cooked in, an amazing junction of culinary and architectural ingenuity that promotes ideal heat conduction and even cooking temperature. There are a bazillion versions of tagine out there—chicken, lamb, beef, goat, vegetable—but what they all have in common is that they're cooked low and slow. This recipe for braised chicken with green olives and lemons in a sauce perfumed with turmeric, saffron, and cilantro is based on one of the most classic tagines (and my favorite). Alas, this recipe is also pretty inauthentic (but undeniably delicious). For one thing, I don't cook mine in a tagine dish. Why? Because I don't have one, so you can stop worrying about whether you can make the dish in your regular-person kitchen. You can. Any wide, shallow pot with a tight-fitting lid will work. Second, people may tell you that preserved lemon is a must in this recipe. I am here to tell you that if you can find preserved lemon in your supermarket or specialty store, its unique sour/bitter/savory flavor will add lovely depth to your tagine, but if you can't find it, you can use regular lemon and all will work out. Third, I always serve a tagine with couscous, which is certainly a Moroccan ingredient but not usually served with a tagine in Morocco, as couscous is its own dish there. You can use bread or rice, if you like, but you're going to want *some* vehicle for mopping up all that yummy, saucy business.

Continued

Serves 4 to 6

3 tablespoons olive oil

2 large yellow onions, sliced

3 garlic cloves, minced

½ teaspoon salt

2 teaspoons ground ginger

1 teaspoon ground turmeric

½ teaspoon crushed saffron threads

1 teaspoon ground cinnamon

Juice of ½ lemon

Rind of 2 small preserved lemons, cut into slivers, or grated zest of 1 large fresh lemon

2 tablespoons chopped fresh parsley

1 small bunch cilantro, coarsely chopped

6 whole chicken leg quarters or 6 drumsticks and 6 thighs

3 tablespoons cracked green olives

1 cup water or chicken stock

1. Heat a tagine or heavy-bottomed, shallow, lidded pan (a Dutch oven works well) over low heat. Add the oil, then the sliced onions. Sprinkle with the garlic, salt, ginger, turmeric, saffron, and cinnamon, followed by the lemon juice and the rind of the preserved lemons (reserve the pulp for another use) *or* the grated zest of one large fresh lemon. Add the parsley and 2 tablespoons of the chopped cilantro and toss the mixture to combine.

2. Arrange the chicken on top of the onion mixture and scatter with the olives. Pour the water or stock into the

pan and bring to a boil. Lower the heat, cover tightly, and simmer gently for 40 to 45 minutes, until the chicken is cooked through.

3. Season to taste and top with the remaining cilantro.

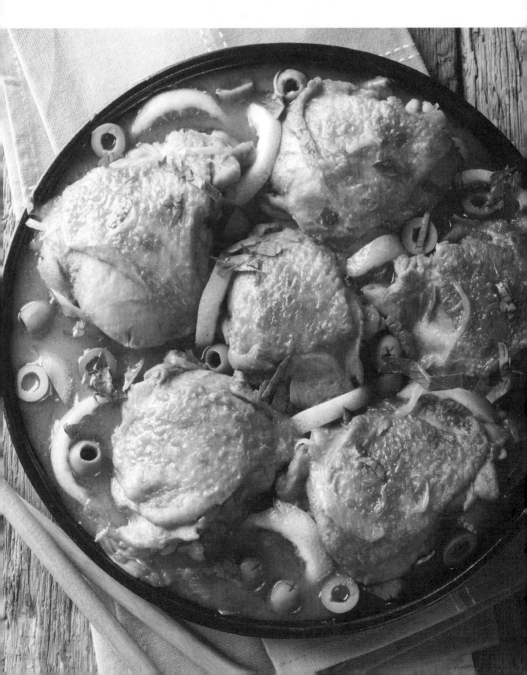

GINGER-SCALLION CHICKEN THIGHS ⓖ

Oh, this chicken. With a perfectly crispy skin, juicy interior, and a sweet-spicy sauce, it hits all the marks. *So* delicious. And, frankly, it's pretty hard to mess up. Relying on my favorite piece of chicken (bone-in, skin-on thighs) with my favorite cooking method, the result is not only a great dish but a solid blueprint for lots and lots of other great dishes down the road. Here, ginger is the flavor star—bright, spicy, and warming—but the cooking method is actually what makes the recipe work, so you could make it the same way but vary the flavoring and still knock it out of the park. (Don't believe me? Check out my Honey Lime Chicken Thighs recipe in *The Honey Companion*—guaranteed déjà vu.) It's simple: You start with the thighs, skin side down in a cold skillet, cook them until they're bronzed and crisp, then blast them in a hot oven until they're perfectly done. Super easy, quick, and reliably tender. You'll have just enough time to pull together some rice and a salad or a green vegetable (and open a bottle of wine?) while they finish in the oven.

Serves 4

¼ cup pure maple syrup
¼ cup fresh lemon or lime juice, or rice vinegar
1 tablespoon soy sauce
2 tablespoons minced fresh ginger

1 garlic clove, minced

2 pounds bone-in, skin-on chicken thighs (4 to 6 thighs)

2 tablespoons olive oil

½ teaspoon salt

Freshly ground black pepper

2 scallions, white and green parts, thinly sliced

1. Arrange a rack in the middle of the oven and preheat the oven to 400°F.

2. Combine the maple syrup, lemon juice, soy sauce, ginger, and garlic in a small bowl. Mix well.

3. Drizzle the chicken thighs with the olive oil and season well with the salt and pepper.

4. Place the thighs, skin side down, in a single layer in a large, cold, cast-iron skillet. Place the skillet over medium heat and cook for 14 to 15 minutes, until the skin is crispy and browned. Turn the chicken and pour the sauce mixture over the thighs.

5. Transfer the skillet to the oven and roast until the chicken reaches an internal temperature of 165°F, about 15 minutes. Garnish with the scallions and serve immediately.

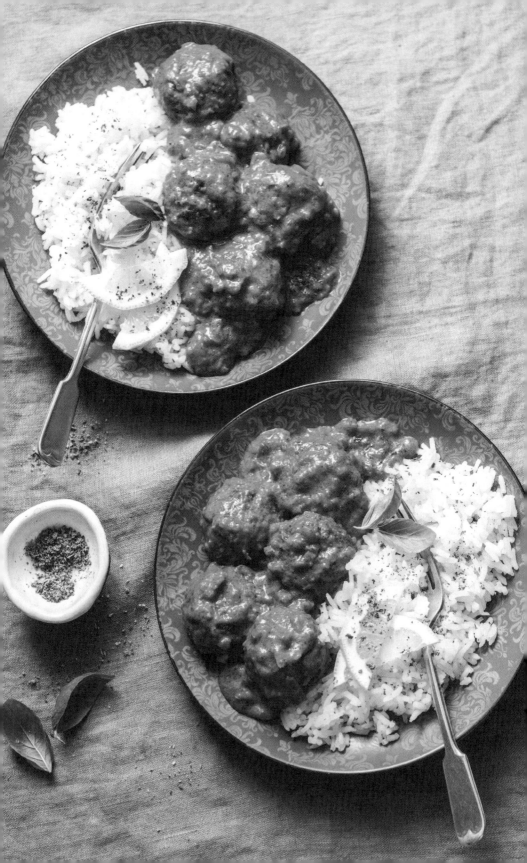

LEMONGRASS AND GINGER MEATBALLS IN COCONUT CURRY BROTH (G)

If the word *meatballs* immediately conjures images of spaghetti and red sauce for you, prepare to experience a serious mind shift—this meal is going to change the way you think about meatballs. Here, ground chicken (or really any ground meat you like) is mixed with a killer roster of bright, Thai-inspired ingredients, including ginger, cilantro, basil, and lemongrass, rolled into bite-sized balls, then bathed in a fragrant broth of coconut milk and yellow curry paste. Served in a bowl with a heap of jasmine rice or a tangle of noodles, this dish is a comfort food experience like no other. Bear in mind, while yellow curry paste is *relatively* mild, it does pack some heat, so feel free to adjust the amount you use to suit your level of spice tolerance.

Serves 4

MEATBALLS:

1 pound ground chicken (or another ground meat, if you prefer)

4 scallions, minced

2 cloves garlic, minced

1 tablespoon grated fresh ginger

1 tablespoon Thai yellow curry paste

Continued

¼ cup panko bread crumbs

1 tablespoon finely chopped fresh cilantro, plus more for serving

1 tablespoon finely chopped fresh basil

1 tablespoon finely chopped lemongrass (tender white part only)

1 teaspoon salt

½ teaspoon freshly ground black pepper

BROTH:

1 tablespoon canola oil

1 tablespoon minced garlic

1 tablespoon minced ginger

2 tablespoons Thai yellow curry paste

Zest of 2 limes

1 cup coconut milk

2 cups chicken or vegetable stock

TO SERVE:

Juice of 2 limes

A few handfuls fresh spinach, mustard greens, or other dark green leaves of your choosing (optional)

Fresh ground black pepper (optional)

1. Adjust the oven rack to the center position and preheat the oven to 375°F.

2. Prepare the meatballs: Place all the meatball ingredients in a large bowl and, using your hands, mix together until blended. Form the meat mixture into 1- to 1½-tablespoon-sized meatballs.

3. Place the balls about an inch apart on a parchment-lined baking sheet. Bake for 15 to 20 minutes, until cooked through.

4. Meanwhile, prepare the broth: Heat the oil in a medium saucepan over medium heat. Add the garlic and ginger and sauté for about 30 seconds, or until fragrant. Add the curry paste and cook for another 30 seconds, then stir in the lime zest, coconut milk, and stock. Bring to a simmer.

5. To assemble: When the meatballs are fully cooked, remove them from the oven and place them in the broth. Toss in the spinach or greens of your choosing (if using) and cook for another 2 to 3 minutes, until they're bright green and wilted. Remove the pan from the heat and stir in the lime juice. Add more black pepper to taste, if desired. Serve.

GARLIC-GINGER MARINATED FLANK STEAK Ⓖ

I don't eat a lot of red meat. In fact, I eat very little red meat. As in, maybe once every couple of months. I'm definitely not a vegetarian, as I eat plenty of fish, eggs, and some poultry, but I do lead a relatively plant-centric existence. This is all partly for health reasons, partly for karmic reasons, and partly for planetary reasons, but mostly it's because I just don't love meat that much. Except every once in a while I *do* decide that I'm in the mood and that I want to splurge on some red meat, in which case I want it to be really, really good. Like. Really. Good. I want it to be a little salty, a little tangy, a little punchy, and definitely beefy. I want it to be this here steak. This recipe makes a whole flank steak, which is either great for entertaining or for generating leftovers, which you'll undoubtedly be happy to have lingering about, because it's excellent served cold as part of a steak salad (think: sliced cucumbers, blanched green beans, julienned peppers, crushed peanuts, cilantro, and lime) or in a sandwich. And if you're more partial to another cut of meat, you can easily use skirt or hanger steak instead.

Serves 6 to 8

1 tablespoon water

¼ cup light or dark brown sugar

1½ tablespoons Asian fish sauce, or more to taste

3 tablespoons fresh lime juice

1 garlic clove, minced

1½ teaspoons fresh ginger, minced

½ teaspoon crushed red pepper flakes

1 whole flank steak, about 2 pounds

Salt

Freshly ground black pepper

1. Combine the water, brown sugar, fish sauce, lime juice, garlic, ginger, and red pepper flakes in a small bowl and stir to combine.

2. Place the flank steak and the marinade in a resealable, gallon-sized plastic bag. Press out the air, seal the bag, and place the steak in the refrigerator to marinate for at least 1 hour and up to 12 hours.

3. Meanwhile, preheat (and clean the grates of) an outdoor grill, indoor grill pan, or oven broiler.

4. Remove the steak from the marinade, season both sides with salt and black pepper, and place on the hot grill. Cook for 3 to 5 minutes per side, depending on the thickness of the meat and your preference for doneness. I like mine medium rare, which is about 125°F and takes less than 4 minutes per side, but you do you.

5. Remove the steak from the grill and allow it to rest for 5 to 10 minutes. Slice the meat very thinly against the grain. Serve.

COCONUT AND RED LENTIL DAL G T

This easy, vegan, gluten-free, dairy-free, flavor-packed Indian-style curry is a great weeknight meal: ready in under 30 minutes and cooked in one pot. What more can one ask of a workweek dinner? The coconut milk makes the dish feel decadent, while the lentils and spices keep it homey yet, somehow, still light and revitalizing. And about those red lentils . . . should you get halfway through the recipe and panic that things have gone terribly wrong because the once teensy, coral-colored lentils have morphed into what can only be described as yellow "mush," rest assured, that's supposed to happen. Unlike black lentils or yellow split peas, red lentils cook down really quickly and become lusciously creamy. Feel free to bulk up the dish by adding whatever vegetables you have around, such as a few handfuls of spinach, sliced carrots, diced sweet potato, or winter squash. Then serve the whole shebang over white or brown rice to round out the meal. Or add a bit more liquid to thin things out and make it more soup-like and less of a stew. Any way you serve it, this one-pot wonder will quickly become a favorite dish.

Serves 6 to 8

Continued

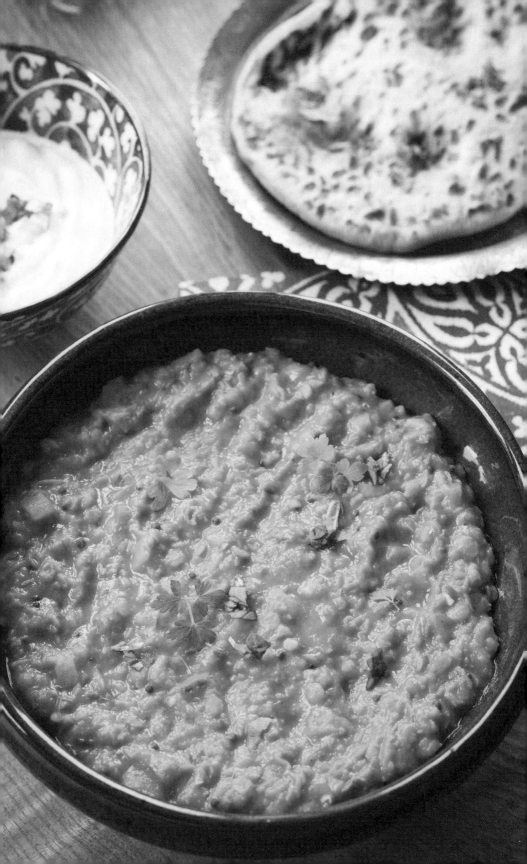

2 tablespoons vegetable oil

1 medium onion, chopped finely

1 tablespoon peeled and finely chopped fresh ginger

2 garlic cloves, minced

1 teaspoon ground cumin

½ teaspoon ground coriander

1 teaspoon ground turmeric

1 teaspoon salt, plus more to serve

¼ teaspoon freshly ground black pepper

1 fresh jalapeño or serrano chile, finely chopped, including seeds (optional)

2 cups water

1½ cups dried red lentils

One 14-ounce can unsweetened coconut milk

2 tomatoes, seeded and chopped

1 cup loosely packed fresh cilantro sprigs

Lime wedges for serving

1. Heat the oil in a heavy, 3½- to 4-quart pot over moderate heat. Add the onion and cook until translucent, about 6 minutes. Add the ginger and garlic and cook for 1 minute. Add the cumin, coriander, turmeric, salt, black pepper, and chile and cook for 1 minute more.

2. Add the water, lentils, and coconut milk. Stir to combine, then simmer, covered, stirring occasionally, for 5 minutes. Stir in the tomatoes and simmer, covered, until the lentils and tomatoes are tender, about 15 minutes.

3. Season with salt and serve with cilantro sprigs and lime wedges.

TURMERIC CAKE WITH HONEY CREAM CHEESE FROSTING Ⓣ

Unexpected as it may seem to see turmeric turn up in a cake recipe, this idea is far from a new one. You see, there's a delicious and very old Lebanese cake called *sfouf*, which is made from semolina flour and turmeric. It is brightly hued, just sweet enough to perfectly complement a cup of coffee or tea, and is perfumed with the unique, earthy, and delicate touch of turmeric that mingles just so with the modest dose of sugar and orange flower water. On the spectrum of baked goods, traditional sfouf sits closer to biscotti and corn bread than a true dessert. This recipe, however, is a riff on the original: it's sweeter, moister, and (with apologies to purists and traditional sfouf lovers) it gets a slathering of decadent honey-kissed cream cheese frosting, which not only places it squarely in the dessert category but makes it perfectly suited to celebrations—just add candles. Perhaps my favorite part of this recipe is the use of tahini (sesame paste) to grease the pan. It's a very common instruction in many traditional sfouf recipes, and I just love how it adds to the unique character and richness of the cake. Of course, you can coat the pans with oil or butter instead and still end up with a showstopper of a treat!

Serves 12

Continued

CAKE:

1 to 2 tablespoons tahini for pan

2½ cups all-purpose flour

4 teaspoons ground turmeric

2 teaspoons baking powder

½ teaspoon salt

12 tablespoons (1½ sticks) unsalted butter, at room temperature

2 cups granulated sugar

3 large eggs

1 cup whole milk

½ teaspoon vanilla extract

1 teaspoon rose water or orange flower water (optional)

FROSTING:

8 ounces cream cheese, at room temperature

4 tablespoons (½ stick) unsalted butter, at room temperature

Pinch of salt

⅓ cup honey, preferably raw

3 to 4 cups powdered sugar

1. Prepare the cake: Preheat the oven to 350°F. Line the bottoms of two 8- or 9-inch round pans with parchment paper and grease the sides with the tahini.

2. Whisk together the flour, turmeric, baking powder, and salt in a bowl. Set aside.

3. Using a separate bowl and a hand mixer or a stand mixer fitted with the paddle attachment, beat the butter and

granulated sugar together until light and fluffy, then add the eggs, one at a time, beating until fully incorporated and the mixture is pale yellow. Add the flour mixture and beat at low speed until just barely mixed. Add the milk, vanilla, and rose water (if using) and beat together on low speed until everything is fully incorporated, scraping down the sides of the bowl as needed.

4. Divide the batter evenly between the prepared pans and bake for 25 to 30 minutes, until the tops spring back slightly when pressed and the cake pulls away from the sides of the pan. Let cool on wire racks for at least 15 minutes, then flip each pan over onto the rack to cool the cakes completely.

5. Prepare the frosting: Combine the cream cheese, butter, salt, and honey in a bowl to mix with a handheld mixer or in a stand mixer fitted with the paddle attachment. Beat until fluffy, 2 to 3 minutes. Gradually add the powdered sugar and beat until smooth, about 1 minute more.

6. Frost and assemble the cake: Place one cake layer on a cake plate or platter. Spread about one-third of the frosting over the layer, all the way to the edge. Place the second layer on top of the first and frost the top and sides of the cake with the remaining frosting.

Note: Unfrosted and wrapped in plastic wrap, the cakes will keep at room temperature for 1 week or frozen for up to 3 months.

ONE-BOWL GINGER APPLE CAKE Ⓖ

Sometimes you need a cake fast. Like, when you suddenly remember a coworker's birthday, or you're invited to a last-minute coffee, or you are just having one of those days when you *need* cake. Need it. Right now! These are times when I imagine a cake mix would come in handy; they come together quickly and there's almost no mess to clean up. I don't really have anything against cake mixes; I just don't like the artificial taste, so I don't use them. Instead, when faced with a cake emergency, I opt for this moist, gooey, no fuss, no muss, gingery apple cake. Like a cake mix, it's literally a dump, stir, pour, and bake undertaking with only nine ingredients, and one mixing bowl, and very little measuring or cleanup. You can use dried ginger in place of the fresh; the flavor won't be quite the same, but it definitely works and will, obviously, save time. Serve this quick-as-a-wink cake plain or with a scoop of ice cream, a dollop of whipped cream, or—my favorite—a schmear of cream cheese.

Serves 8 to 10

½ cup vegetable oil, plus more to oil pan

2 large eggs

1¾ cups sugar

2 teaspoons ground cinnamon

1 tablespoon grated fresh ginger, or 1 teaspoon ground

6 medium apples, peeled and thinly sliced

2 teaspoons baking soda

¼ teaspoon salt

2 cups all-purpose flour

1. Preheat the oven to 350°F. Oil a 9-by-13-inch baking pan with a little vegetable oil.

2. Mix together the oil, eggs, sugar, cinnamon, and ginger in a large bowl. Add the apple slices and toss to coat. Sprinkle the baking soda and salt over the apple mixture, then add the flour and stir just until no raw flour is visible in the batter.

3. Pour into the prepared pan and bake in the center of the oven until the cake is golden brown and a toothpick inserted into the center comes out clean, 40 to 50 minutes. Remove from the oven and let cool for 10 minutes before serving.

SWEET AND SPICY CANDIED GINGER ⓖ

We are a family that takes a lot of long-distance car rides. For many holidays and other family functions, we pack up our car full of toys, snacks, games, and other assorted tricks and tools for keeping our kids entertained. Oh, and suitcases. If there's room. It can be a long ride. One year, what should have been a four-hour drive took us nine hours and 37 minutes. All of which is to say that I am a very experienced car-based flight attendant. I've got a pretty good system for stuck-in-traffic emergency preparedness, including entertainment, sustenance, side-of-the-road bathroom needs, and motion sickness. As such, my kit always includes a stash of this homemade candied ginger, which solves snacking-related problems as well as motion sickness, as ginger is one of the best anti-nausea treatments around. Spicy, sweet, easy to make, and *so* much less expensive to DIY than it is to buy, you're going to feel so silly for not having made your own before. When we're not in the car, I bake with it (love it chopped and added to cookies!) or serve it on its own as a little after-dinner treat for party guests. It's lovely just as is or, even better, dipped in dark chocolate.

Makes about 1 pound ginger

1 pound fresh ginger, peeled and sliced as thinly as possible
4 cups sugar, plus more for coating the ginger slices
4 cups water
Pinch of salt

1. Place the ginger slices in a large saucepan and add enough water to fully cover them. Simmer, uncovered, over medium-high heat for 20 minutes. Drain.

2. Mix together the sugar, 4 cups of water, a pinch of salt, and drained ginger in the same saucepan and cook until a candy thermometer reads 225°F or the liquid thickens and becomes syrupy, 20 to 30 minutes.

3. Remove the pan from the heat and allow it to stand for about an hour. Strain the ginger through a colander or fine-mesh sieve set over a large bowl to catch the syrup (use it to make cocktails or sweeten your tea!), allowing it to drip for a good 30 minutes or so.

4. Toss the drained slices in additional sugar. Shake off any excess sugar and spread the ginger slices on a parchment-lined baking sheet or wire rack. Let dry for at least 3 hours or overnight, until they're quite dry.

5. Store in an airtight container at room temperature in a dry place and away from direct sunlight. Your candy will keep for several months.

AMAZING NO-CHURN TURMERIC AND MANGO SORBET Ⓣ

The people in my house are big fans of frozen treats. Ice cream, ice pops, sorbet, granita, Italian ice . . . they love it all. When my kids say, "Mommy, can we have a treat?" they don't usually mean "Can we have a cookie?" or "Can we have a piece of cake?" Generally, what they're asking for (and what my frozen-treat-fanatic husband has trained them to think of as *real* dessert) is something from the freezer. As such, I have been known to churn some lavish and involved concoctions in the ice cream maker for such special occasions as birthdays and Father's Day and when we've gone peach or berry picking as a family. But for everyday purposes, when I'm not interested in serving them a ton of sugar and when I'm short on time, I love the genius of a no-churn recipe. Here, you combine frozen mango, turmeric, and a few other very simple ingredients to achieve sorbet that's fast; low in added sugar; packed with fresh, vibrant flavor; gorgeous to look at; and a great way to squeeze a little more turmeric into your day. The beauty is that you don't even need an ice cream maker to concoct this delicious icy treat!

Makes about 2 cups sorbet

12 ounces frozen mango chunks

1 teaspoon grated lime zest

Juice of ½ lime

2 teaspoons ground turmeric, or 2 tablespoons grated fresh

⅔ cup water

Pinch of salt

5 tablespoons sugar, or more to taste

1. Put the frozen mango chunks into a high-speed blender or food processor fitted with a metal blade. Add the remaining incredients.

2. Pulse and process until the ingredients are completely blended and resemble soft-serve ice cream. Eat immediately or transfer the mixture to a container and freeze 2 to 3 hours, until firm enough to scoop.

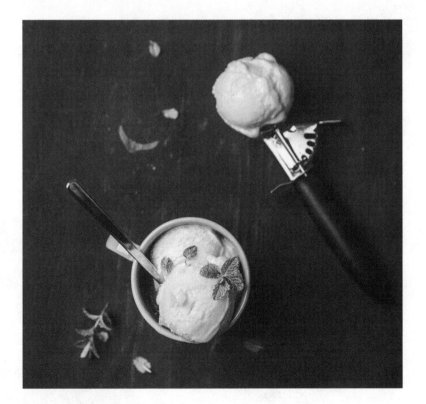

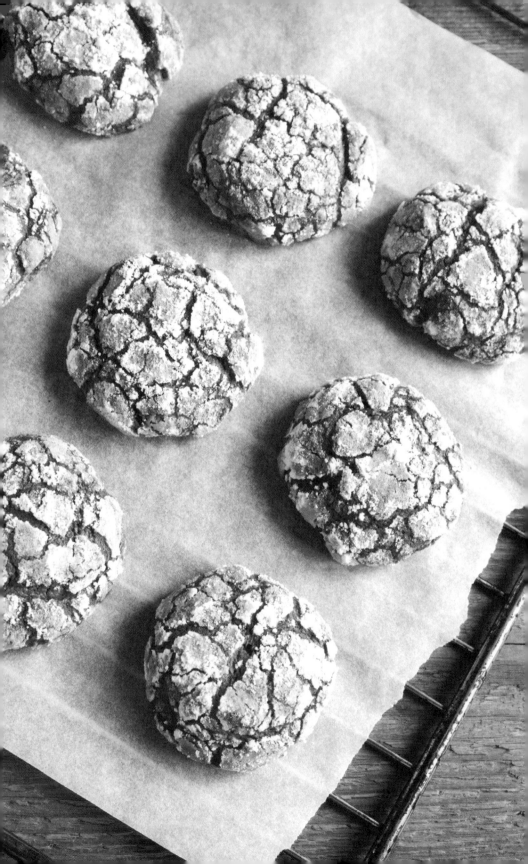

CHEWY TRIPLE-GINGER CHOCOLATE COOKIES Ⓖ

Once upon a time, in our early dating days, my husband and I rented a car and took an adorable little day trip to go apple picking in "the country." We were in that flirty, wooing stage of our courtship, and I decided to try to impress him with a batch of homemade cookies for the drive. I'd learned he was partial to a chewy cookie, but I wanted to make something sort of out of the box. Standard-issue chocolate chip cookies, while never a bad choice, were just too pedestrian for the impact I wanted to make; after all, I was still trying to snag this guy! I ended up finding a version of this recipe somewhere on the Internet and thought it would be perfect: sweet, spicy, and interesting enough to be memorable. I tweaked it quite a bit to include chopped crystallized ginger in addition to the ground and fresh ginger, a heftier dose of chocolate, and a crunchy coating of turbinado sugar. In the end, triple the ginger, double the chocolate . . . slam dunk! So, to all the single ladies and gentlemen out there, while I can't say for sure that these were the cookies that sealed the deal, my husband still remembers eating them in the car that day and asks me to make them often. If you've got your eye on someone special, these beauties are probably worth a try.

Makes about 3 dozen cookies

Continued

1½ cups all-purpose flour

½ cup unsweetened cocoa powder

1 teaspoon baking soda

½ teaspoon kosher salt

1¼ teaspoons ground ginger

1 teaspoon ground cinnamon

¼ teaspoon ground cloves

¼ teaspoon freshly ground black pepper

¼ teaspoon ground nutmeg

8 ounces good-quality dark chocolate, chopped into ¼-inch chunks

8 tablespoons (1 stick) unsalted butter

1 tablespoon peeled and grated fresh ginger

1 cup dark brown sugar

¼ cup unsulfured molasses

2 large eggs

⅓ cup coarsely chopped crystalized ginger

⅓ cup turbinado sugar, or another coarse sugar, for coating cookies

1. Whisk together the flour, cocoa powder, baking soda, salt, and spices in a medium bowl; set aside.

2. Melt 4 ounces of the chopped chocolate with the butter in a small, heatproof bowl set over a pan of simmering water, or microwave in 30-second intervals on HIGH until melted.

3. Transfer the chocolate mixture to a large mixing bowl to use with a handheld mixer, or the bowl of an electric mixer fitted with the paddle attachment. Add the fresh ginger, brown sugar, molasses, and eggs and mix until combined. Gradually mix in the flour mixture. Fold in the remaining chocolate chunks and crystallized ginger. Cover the bowl with plastic wrap and refrigerate for 1 hour.

4. Scoop the dough into ½-inch balls and place 2 inches apart on parchment-lined baking sheets. Refrigerate for 20 minutes, then roll in turbinado sugar. Meanwhile, preheat the oven to 350°F.

5. Bake the cookies, rotating the pan at about the 6-minute point, until they flatten and their surfaces begin to crack, 10 to 12 minutes. *Do not overbake!* Remove from the oven and cool on a wire rack. Serve and live happily ever after.

6. The cookies can be stored in an airtight container at room temperature for up to 3 days.

HEALING
TREATMENTS

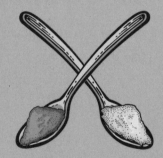

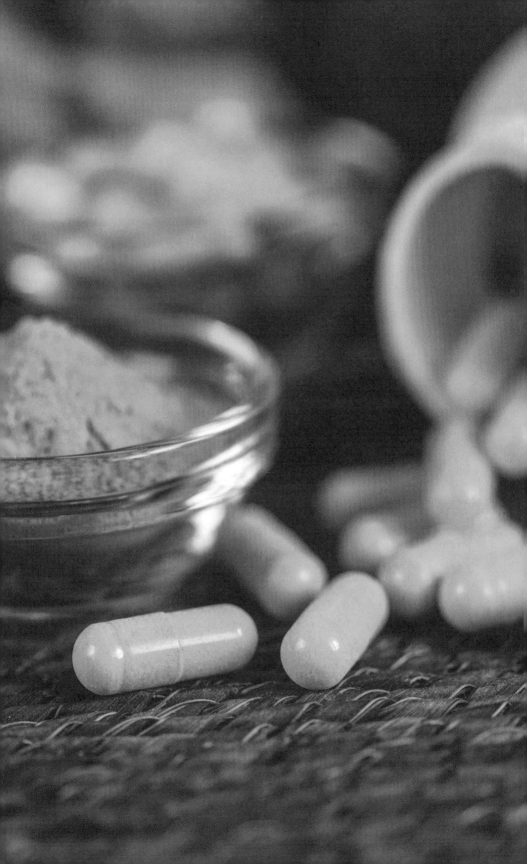

IMMUNITY-BOOSTING SHOT Ⓖ

Believe it or not, "Wanna do a shot?" is a common inquiry in my kitchen during the early morning mad dash to get everyone off to school and work. While I do confess that amid half-made lunches, tantruming kids, a spilled smoothie, and a missing sneaker, I have more than once fantasized about a leisurely happy hour with a lovely glass of wine, the kind of shot I'm talking about isn't boozy at all. It's a small, potent dose of ginger that my husband and I rely on to keep ourselves in fighting shape or, at the very least, clear of the colds and other illnesses we simply don't have time to deal with. A ginger shot—which is more or less pure ginger juice—is a direct delivery of all the benefits of ginger. Straight up. With antioxidants to fight free radicals and toxins in your body and anti-inflammatory properties that will aid your recovery if you're already knocked down by something, this shot is a lifesaver. I add lemon juice for an extra dose of vitamin C and to cut the heat of the ginger a little. Even so, it isn't for the faint of heart. This stuff is intense. If you like, you can add a little bit of maple syrup to ease up on the heat even more, but remember it's a shot, not a sipper, so toss it back and get on with your day. And if your version of "Wanna do a shot?" does mean what it's *supposed* to mean, you can always turn to this wellness shot the next day to help you ease back into things.

Makes 8 to 10 treatments

2 large knobs ginger (about 4 ounces), peeled and chopped roughly

1 cup fresh lemon juice (from 3 to 4 lemons)

Pure maple syrup (optional)

1. Place the ginger and lemon juice in a high-speed blender or juicer. Process until very smooth.

2. Pass the mixture through a fine-mesh sieve, pushing the pulp against the screen with the back of a spoon or rubber spatula to squeeze out as much liquid as possible.

3. Store the reserved juice in the refrigerator for up to a week. Drink 1 to 2 ounces daily, sweetened with maple syrup to taste, if desired.

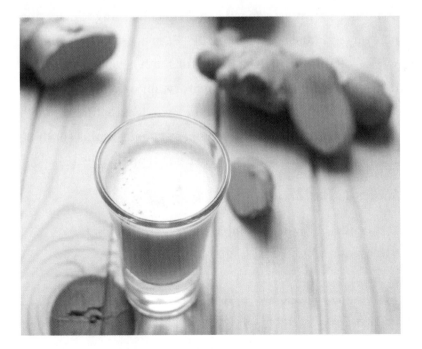

COUGH SUPPRESSANT Ⓣ

What's worse than a nagging, hacking cough that disrupts your daily groove? The night cough, that's what! You know the one I'm talking about. The cough that shows up just as you start to think you're getting over a cold or the flu. The one that sneaks up, like clockwork, just as evening sets in, even though you've barely coughed all day. The one that is determined to keep you up all freaking night. Yeah, *that* one. Well, watch out, Night Cough! Here comes a simple, natural remedy so full of powerful nutrients, it'll kick you and the rest of those nasty cold symptoms to the curb. The whole lot of you! Here comes honey—KAPOW!—a well-researched and documented natural cough suppressant that's packed with antiviral, antibacterial, and other soothing properties to help calm things down. And now turmeric and black pepper, like Batman—BOOM!—and his sidekick Robin—BAM!—a powerful combo, working together to bring even more anti-inflammatory, antioxidant, and antiviral ammo to your system. Next time you feel that night cough (or any cough) creep in, make yourself a mug of this soothing sipper and prepare for victory. See ya, Night Cough!

Makes 1 treatment

1 cup milk (coconut, almond, dairy, or any other kind)

¾ teaspoon ground turmeric

¼ teaspoon ground cinnamon

1 tablespoon raw honey

Pinch of freshly ground black pepper

1. Put all the ingredients in a small saucepan or microwave-able mug and stir to combine.

2. Heat over medium-high heat for 2 to 3 minutes, stirring occasionally, or microwave on HIGH for about 1 minute, until the mixture is very hot but not boiling.

3. Stir again and sip slowly, stirring and swirling as you go to keep the spices from settling at the bottom of the mug.

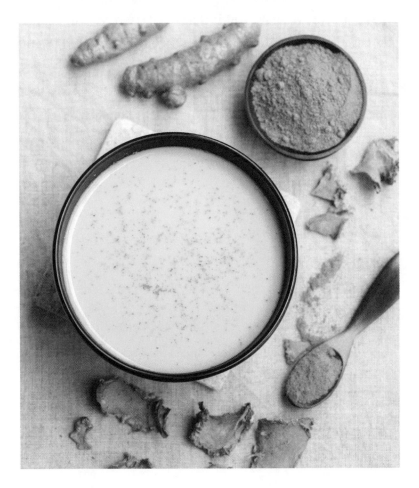

EXTREMELY ATTRACTIVE
SORE THROAT GARGLE Ⓖ

Gargling is a simple, highly effective, time-tested way to kill germs and soothe a sore throat. It also looks and sounds extremely attractive! Mmm-hmmm. Be sure that when you gargle and spit you do so in front of your significant other or, better yet, someone you've just started dating, because it's super sexy. Well, no. But it *is* a super effective way to heal and calm a raw, scratchy, irritated throat. In addition to ginger, this potent solution includes apple cider vinegar—great for killing bacteria and loosening phlegm—as well as sea salt, which reduces inflammation, clears mucus, and helps fight off bacteria in the throat, plus raw honey, which coats the throat and brings flavor and even more antiseptic firepower. Make a fresh batch of this stuff every time you need to gargle, which you should do a few times a day until your symptoms subside, because you don't want to run the risk of having bacteria set up camp in a glass you've left hanging around. Gross.

Makes 1 treatment

½ cup hot water

1 tablespoon raw, organic apple cider vinegar

1 teaspoon raw honey

¼ teaspoon sea salt

½ teaspoon ground ginger

1. Combine all the ingredients in a mug or glass. Stir to combine, making sure to dissolve the honey.

2. Sip some of the mixture, gargle for several seconds, then spit. Repeat with the rest of the solution, making sure to give a wink and flash your best "come hither" look at whomever catches you in the act.

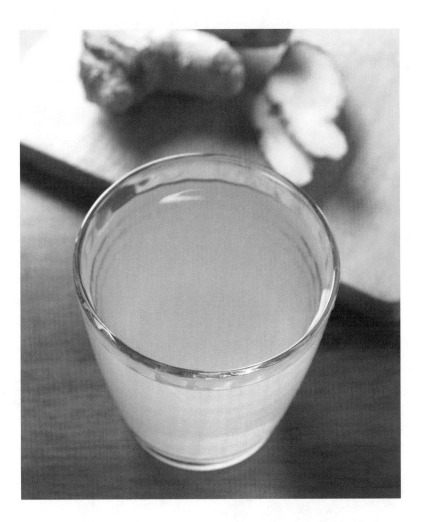

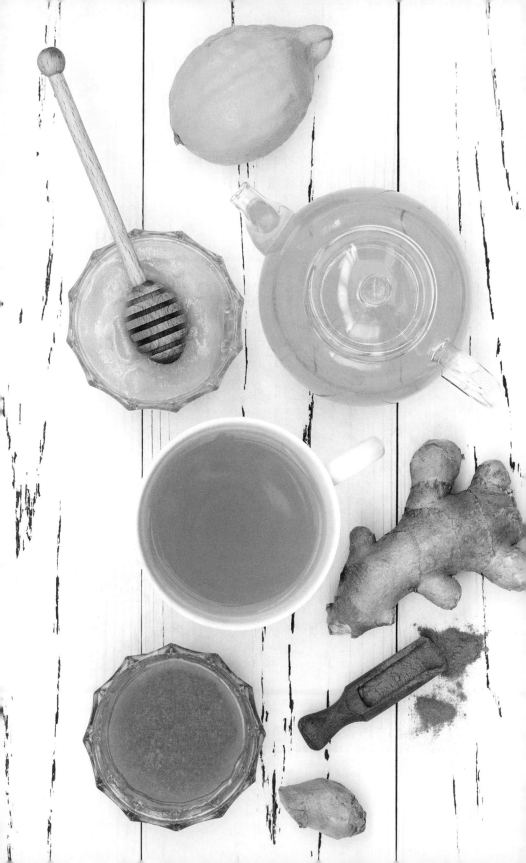

COLD-FIGHTING WELLNESS TONIC Ⓖ Ⓣ

Here's a simple, effective, and all-natural way to DIY back into fighting shape when you're sniffling, sneezing, coughing, and otherwise battling a cold. With a squad of anti-inflammatory and immunity-boosting ingredients, such as herbs, spices and vitamin C–rich citrus, this wellness tonic—a nutrient-dense powerhouse that packs a punch—will stop your cold in its tracks. Like a supercharged multivitamin, this elixir works best if taken with a little fat (say, a fried egg or a spoonful of peanut butter) to help your body absorb all those nutrients. Buckwheat honey is said to be particularly effective in calming cold symptoms. If you don't have buckwheat honey (or don't care for the strong flavor of it), no problem; any good-quality raw honey will provide health benefits.

Makes 1 treatment

¼ cup fresh orange juice

¼ cup fresh lemon juice

One ½-inch piece fresh ginger, grated

One ½-inch piece fresh turmeric, grated, or ½ teaspoon
  ground

2 teaspoons buckwheat honey

Pinch of freshly ground black pepper

Place all the ingredients in a small jar. Stir or shake gently to combine. If desired, pass the mixture through a fine-mesh sieve to remove the pulp. Sip.

COLD AND FLU SOOTHER Ⓖ

I freely admit that each year in late fall, after school starts and the weather starts to turn, I begin to obsess and fret a little (*Really, Suzy? A little?*)—okay, a lot—about cold and flu season. I become a handwashing tyrant, which explains why everyone in my house ends up with skin like a crocodile's halfway into winter. (And this, my friends, is why we keep a healthy stash of homemade lotion bars all over the house; check out my book *The Honey Companion* for the fun and easy recipe.) I carry a pack of disinfectant wipes in my bag and use them to wipe down shopping carts, and I change the towels in my house so often they almost march themselves to the laundry room after a single use. Alas, my neurotic behavior is always for naught, as at least one icky bug inevitably makes its way through our house before too long. And so, I turn to this fantastic remedy—a mix of fresh lemon, ginger, and raw honey—to soothe and fight whatever's knocked us down. The lemon, high in vitamin C, boosts immunity. Antiseptic and antiviral ginger not only kills germs but also encourages perspiration, which is super helpful if you're dealing with a fever. And raw honey not only soothes a sore throat and suppresses coughs naturally but has powerful germ-fighting properties to help you get over an illness quickly. Also, this soother is delicious. I like to think ahead and have a batch ready and waiting in the fridge so that, at the first sign of a cold, I can just scoop out a few tablespoons, add hot water, and sip away the sniffles.

Makes about 1 cup soother

Continued

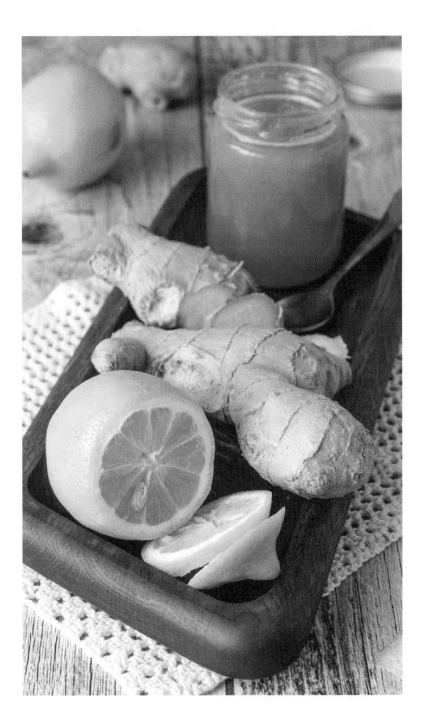

1 cup raw honey

2 lemons, sliced

One 1-inch piece fresh ginger, sliced

1. Pack a pint-sized mason jar or other lidded container with the lemon, ginger, and honey, alternating layers of each.

2. Screw on the lid tightly and place the jar in the refrigerator. Chill for at least 12 hours to allow all the ingredients to meld. You will likely end up with sort of a loose jelly, though, depending on the juiciness of your lemons, the mixture may turn somewhat runny—no problem either way!

3. To use: Scoop 1 to 2 teaspoons of the infused honey into a mug of warm water and drink immediately.

CHERRY-GINGER ELECTROLYTE POPS Ⓖ

About a year ago, we went through a phase in our house wherein my kids brought home a new and different illness pretty much every other week. The flu, colds, a stomach thing . . . you name it, we gave it a try. So, as one does in the face of fevers, congestion, and dehydrating tummy troubles, I tried my best to push fluids and keep those kiddos hydrated. But want to know what's really hard? Getting sick kids to drink fluids. I'd bust out all the fun and fancy cups and straws, offer sugary juices, warm beverages; I'd wear funny hats; I even tried to teach them old college drinking games. And then I'd beg. But no dice. Finally, I started stocking those colorful freezer pops made from electrolyte solution (and a whole bunch of freaky artificial junk) that, naturally, my kids loved. *Damn you, Red No. 40!* After a while, though, I just couldn't keep pumping my sick and pathetic little ones with all those food dyes, added sugars, and fake flavors. So, if ice pops were the answer, I was going to make an ice pop that would actually help them get better. A combination of hydrating coconut water, stomach-soothing ginger, and electrolyte-replacing salt would do the trick. As for flavor, my kids like cherry ice pops, so I went with cherry juice (make sure it's the unsweetened kind, which has shown to raise melatonin and help kids sleep), but feel free to sub in any whole fruit or juice you think will be a winner in your house.

Continued

And just as these babies can help hydrate and soothe little ones who are under the weather, they are a friend to the hungover, too. *Ahem.* Speaking of drinking games . . .

Makes 4 to 8 pops, depending on size

⅓ cup unsweetened tart cherry juice

1 tablespoon fresh lemon juice

½ to 1 teaspoon grated fresh ginger

1 cup raw coconut water

1 to 2 tablespoons pure maple syrup

⅛ teaspoon sea salt

1. Combine all the ingredients in a blender. Process until smooth.

2. Carefully pour the liquid into ice pop molds and freeze until solid.

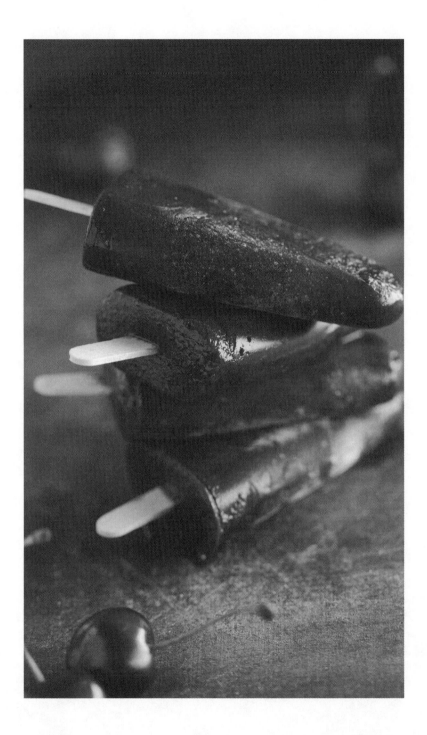

DIY STY TREATMENT (T)

If you suffer from the occasional sty, then you know just how uncomfortable, irritating, and painful they can be. A sty, for the fortunate and uninitiated, is an annoying and surprisingly painful red bump that appears on the eyelid when an oil gland gets clogged and then becomes infected. Those suckers show up right on the eyelid—and I mean, really, is there a worse place?—where they can last up to a few weeks. Turmeric, however, with its powerful antibacterial and anti-inflammatory properties, can help ease the pain and make the sty go away faster. (No matter what, do not try to squeeze the pus from the sty. This can cause the infection to spread to other areas of the eye. Also, it's sooooo gross!) To help prevent sties, make it a habit to *always* wash your hands before touching the skin around your eyes.

Makes 1 treatment

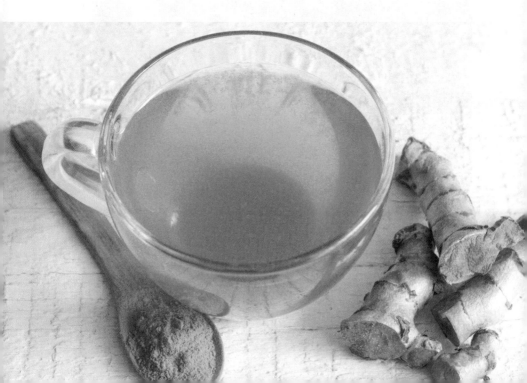

2 teaspoons ground turmeric

1 cup hot water

1. Mix the turmeric and hot water in a small bowl or mug.

2. When the mixture is cool enough to touch to skin but still quite hot, dip a cotton ball into the mixture and, with your eye closed, apply it to the sty. Press down gently and allow the compress to remain on the eye for 10 minutes.

3. Repeat, using a fresh cotton ball, up to five times per day.

HOMEMADE BURN SOOTHER ⓣ

There are two kinds of burns: solid burns, as in real zingers, as in "We have two dinner options in our house—take it or leave it!" Yes, burrrn. And bad burns, as in the kind you get when you have a run-in with a curling iron or an oven rack or even an hour too long in the sun. Ouch. Most minor burns can be treated at home, though if you have blistered or severely injured skin, seek medical attention ASAP to be sure you get the right treatment. For minor burns, after lowering the skin's temperature with cool compresses or ice cubes wrapped in a soft cloth, soothe and heal singed skin with this powerful turmeric treatment.

Makes about ½ cup soother

½ cup aloe vera gel
2 tablespoons coconut oil
1 teaspoon ground turmeric

1. Combine all the ingredients in a small jar or container with a tight-fitting lid. Store the salve in a cool, dark place for up to 3 months.

2. Apply to minor scrapes and burns a few times a day until healed.

ANTISEPTIC FOR CUTS AND SCRAPES Ⓖ

The next time you have a minor cut or scrape on your skin, rub a slice of fresh ginger on it. (Common sense alert: Note the use of the word *minor*! Serious wounds need to be seen by a doctor.) Sure, it may sound a little scary and painful, but trust me. You see, ginger has really strong antiseptic properties, which makes it a great agent for helping heal cuts and abrasions. Plus, gingerol, one of its active ingredients, keeps infections away while improving circulation and encouraging cell regeneration. Isn't that pretty much everything you want when faced with a little skin wound—to keep it clean and to encourage healing? That's it. That's the stuff. As for the pain, remember what it feels like to douse a skinned knee with rubbing alcohol or hydrogen peroxide? *Yowza.* Ginger is a walk in the park!

Makes 1 treatment

1 slice fresh ginger
Waterproof adhesive bandage

1. Wash the wound with clean water.

2. Gently rub the ginger slice directly on the affected area for 5 to 10 seconds. Cover the injury with a waterproof adhesive bandage.

3. Change the dressing daily until the injury is completely healed.

WOUND DISINFECTANT Ⓣ

I read a statistic recently that made me laugh out loud. Apparently, 90 percent of childhood injuries are preventable. The subsequent advice was to keep knives, nails, scissors, and tools locked away and out of children's reach. Hilarious! Yeah, because loose nails are my biggest problem, right? Want to hear the most recent injury that happened at my house? Skinned, bloodied knees from running full steam ahead on the sidewalk while wearing polka-dot rain boots. On the wrong feet. In the sun. Preventable? Sure, *you* try having that conversation with a fiercely independent, fashion-conscious preschooler. Also, note that all sharp objects were locked up at the time. What I'm trying to say is that cuts, scrapes, and minor injuries are a simple fact of life; sooner or later you're going to cut your hand while slicing watermelon/snag your arm on a metal fence/skin your knee after slipping on a piece of sidewalk chalk someone left on the driveway. (All *totally* hypothetical.) The point is you want to be prepared, and having this simple wound treatment on hand to disinfect, soothe, and prevent infection in those inevitable minor cuts and scrapes is certainly a step in the right direction. After locking up your loose nails, of course.

Makes 1 treatment

1 to 2 teaspoons ground turmeric (more for larger wounds)

¼ to ½ teaspoon water

1. Gently wash the affected area with clean, warm water.

2. Mix together the turmeric and water to make a thick paste.

3. With *clean* hands, apply the paste gently to the affected area. Once you've covered the infected area, place an adhesive bandage (Princess variety optional), rolled gauze, or gauze held in place with paper tape over the wound.

4. Change the dressing at least once a day, applying more turmeric paste as necessary, until the wound is healed.

Note: This treatment is for minor cuts and scrapes only. You need to seek *immediate* medical attention if the cut is very deep and/or won't stop bleeding after applying moderate pressure for several minutes, the injured person has not had a tetanus shot within 5 to 10 years, or the cut is from a human or animal bite.

SPRAINED MUSCLE TREATMENT Ⓣ

Sprains are really common injuries, especially if you happen to be a particularly active person, an athlete, and/or a klutz like me. An estimated 25,000 people sprain an ankle every single day—that's how common it is. When a sprain happens, ligaments, often in the ankle, wrist, or knee, have been overstretched (or, in severe cases, torn), usually resulting in instant pain, swelling, and bruising. It's important to seek medical attention right away if you injure yourself and have those symptoms, so you can rule out a broken bone. But once a sprain is diagnosed, you can use this natural remedy to reduce swelling and support other treatments prescribed by your health-care provider. Just remember that you may be sporting a pretty, yellow temporary tattoo while using the treatment. Think of it as a fashion statement!

Makes 1 treatment

1 teaspoon table salt

2 teaspoons ground turmeric

1 to 2 teaspoons water

1. Combine the salt and turmeric with enough water to make a spreadable paste. Apply to the injured muscle and wrap it in a cloth (an old one that you don't mind staining).

2. Leave the paste on for 30 to 40 minutes, then rinse. Repeat one or two times a day until the pain and swelling subside.

Note: To remove turmeric stains from the skin, just dip a cotton ball in coconut oil and rub, rub, rub!

GINGER COMPRESS FOR JOINT PAIN AND MUSCLE STRAIN Ⓖ

I know that exercise is highly beneficial and very necessary for both physical and mental well-being. And there's nothing quite like a really good workout, but I'd be lying if I said I didn't find the often accompanying aches and pains to be kind of annoying. I mean, after all that hard work! Of course, I understand that it has to do with lactic acid buildup and microscopic muscle tears and a whole bunch of other science-y mumbo jumbo, but it just seems kind of unfair for our body to freak out on us like that! I do find, however, that giving sore muscles a little TLC in the form of a ginger compress is a good way to make peace with my body. Give this natural compress a try the next time you've overdone a workout, twisted or turned the wrong way, are fed up with chronic pain from such conditions as arthritis, or feel that you might be coming down with the flu, rather than reach for your usual over-the-counter meds to treat your aches and pains. It'll stimulate circulation, which will in turn relieve pain, relax your muscles, reduce stiffness, and even help release toxins. And don't forget to forgive your body for freaking out a little bit from time to time—it's hard work being you!

Makes 1 treatment

½ cup grated fresh ginger

2 cups water

Bring the ginger and water to a boil in a small saucepan over high heat. Lower the heat to medium-low and simmer for 5 minutes. Remove from the heat and steep the mixture for 15 minutes, then soak a cloth in the liquid. When cool enough to handle but still quite warm, apply to the affected area until cool. Repeat as needed.

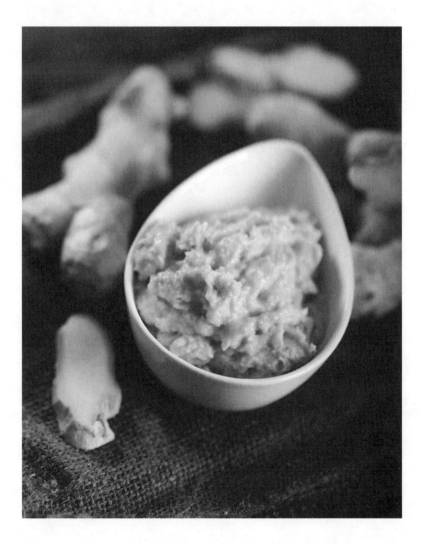

MIGRAINE REMEDY ⒼⓉ

When you suffer from migraines, the search for relief can be frustratingly endless. Migraines are not your run-of-the-mill headache; they're another kind of beast entirely. They can last for a few hours, even a few days, and generate serious, throbbing pain that may cause nausea, pain behind the eyes, sensitivity to light, and/or blurred vision. It's not always clear what brings on these day-wrecking headaches—diet, stress, and hormones are among the often-suspected culprits—but research shows that inflammation in the brain is a known trigger. Prescription drugs and over-the-counter painkillers can sometimes provide relief, but they often come with side effects, such as fatigue and dizziness, not to mention, in the case of opioids, the risk of addiction. If you're trying to reduce your dependence on medication, avoid side effects, or save money, this home remedy may help. The recipe makes a paste that you'll use for tea whenever you're hit with a migraine. Store it in the fridge, and you'll have it at the ready next time you feel one brewing. Just remember, it's always a good idea to consult with your health-care provider before treating any chronic health problems on your own.

Makes about 1¼ cups paste

2½ tablespoons ground turmeric, or more to taste

1½ teaspoons freshly ground black pepper

1 cup raw honey

2 tablespoons ground ginger (optional, but a good idea if you
experience nausea with your headaches)

1. To make the paste: Combine all the ingredients in a jar or
   container with a tight-fitting lid. Stir to blend into a paste.
   (Heating the honey slightly in a microwave for about 10
   seconds makes it easier to incorporate.) The paste keeps
   for *ages* if stored away from direct sunlight and heat.

2. To make tea: Stir 1 to 2 teaspoons of the paste into a cup of
   hot water. Make a cup every few hours, depending on the
   duration of your migraine.

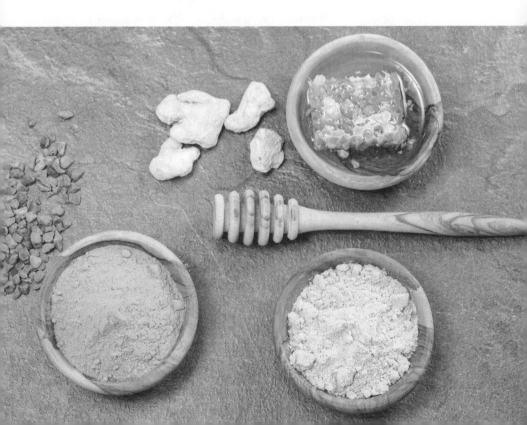

BREATH FRESHENER Ⓖ

It really is amazing how the little things, small indulgences, can make a such a difference in our otherwise bonkers lives. For my husband, it's soap. A few years ago, he declared that he would buy himself only fancy soap and has since walked around happier and smelling like "pine tar" or "charcoal" or "bourbon-tobacco manliness." It's a good thing—everyday luxuries are important, and the guy really enjoys a good shower experience. For me, it's an Italian brand of ridiculously expensive toothpaste. My favorite is its ginger-flavored one. *I know, right?* Ginger sounds like an odd flavor departure for toothpaste (and it did to me, too, but because of the way my brain is wired, it's *exactly* why I had to try it!). But it turns out that ginger is not only refreshing and delicious, it's also scientifically proven to freshen breath! Studies have shown that a compound in ginger—[6]-gingerol—actually stimulates an enzyme in our saliva that breaks down the stinky business in our mouth, kicking bad breath to the curb. So, after I brush with my schmancy toothpaste, or anytime I'm sporting some dragon breath, I like to keep the ginger party pumping with this easy, spicy, gets-the-job-done-right DIY mouth rinse. Ginger, fresh mint, and cinnamon combine to create an anti-inflammatory, antibacterial, fresh-tasting rinse that swishes bad breath right away.

Makes about 3 cups freshener

One 2-inch knob fresh ginger, thinly sliced

½ teaspoon ground cinnamon

⅔ cup packed fresh mint leaves

3 cups water

1. Combine all the ingredients in a medium saucepan. Bring the mixture to a boil, then lower the heat and simmer for anywhere from 20 to 45 minutes, bearing in mind that the longer it simmers, the more intense the flavor will be.

2. Remove from the heat and allow it to cool slightly. Strain the mixture through a fine-mesh sieve into a glass jar or bottle. Allow to cool completely, then store in the refrigerator for up to 3 weeks.

DRY MOUTH REMEDY Ⓖ

Here's a cool word you might not know: *xerostomia*. It means "dry mouth," and if you've ever dealt with it, you know what a bummer it can be to have your mouth somewhat resemble the Sahara. Experiencing dry mouth can be super uncomfortable and may make it hard to talk or swallow, cause cracking at the corners of your lips, and/or a give you a burning sensation on your tongue. There are lots of reasons why you might experience dry mouth, with causes ranging from certain diseases to side effects from medications to vitamin deficiencies to dehydration. The good news is that ginger, which is known to stimulate saliva production, can help you alleviate the discomfort associated with dry mouth. Try sipping this soothing tea two or three times a day consistently for a week or so, and you should experience gradual improvement. If not, see a physician or dentist for consultation and care.

Makes 1 treatment

One 1-inch knob fresh ginger, sliced
1 cup water
Raw honey

Combine the ginger and water in a small saucepan and bring to a boil. Lower the heat and simmer for 2 to 5 minutes. Strain the tea into a mug and add honey to taste.

DIGESTIVE AID ⓖ

You know how your mom used to give you ginger ale when you were home sick from school? There's a reason for that! Ginger is a superstar at settling the stomach. Not only that—thanks to phenolic compounds, including gingerol, it stimulates digestion and aids in transporting body fluids. So, the next time you overindulge or feel that your digestive system requires a bit of calming or de-bloating or is otherwise in need of support, stir up this quick and soothing recipe. I always make it with sparkling water, but I'm a carbonation junkie. If you don't find bubbles soothing, feel free to use still water instead.

Makes 1 treatment

1 teaspoon grated fresh ginger

1 teaspoon fresh lemon juice, lime juice, or raw apple cider vinegar

Sweetener of your choice, to taste (optional)

Water (flat or fizzy)

Combine the ginger, citrus juice or vinegar, and sweetener (if using) in a glass. Stir well to combine. Add ice, if desired, and fill the glass with flat or fizzy water. Gently stir the mixture, then allow the ginger bits to settle to the bottom of the glass. Sip slowly.

DANDRUFF TREATMENT Ⓣ

On the list of beauty-related bummers, dandruff—the condition where your scalp is super flaky and often itchy—is right up there with oily skin and bacne (back acne.) Hormone imbalances, autoimmune diseases, or an overgrowth of the fungus *Malassezia* on the scalp can all lead to seborrheic dermatitis, an overreaction to naturally occurring yeast, a.k.a. dandruff. But no matter the root cause (get it?), you're going to want soothing relief and a way to eliminate those embarrassing flakes. Although over-the-counter dandruff shampoos are easy to find, they're full of chemicals and, according to some studies, may even lose efficacy over time. Your best bet? A combination of coconut oil and turmeric, both of which have natural antifungal properties to restore balance to your scalp.

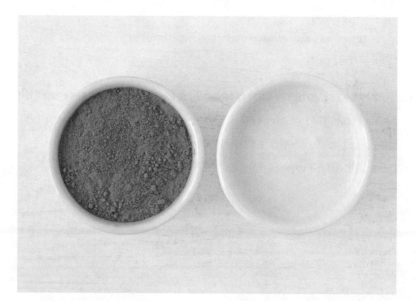

Coconut oil will moisturize and soothe irritated skin, and antiseptic turmeric helps to quell inflammation, giving you nearly instant relief. Just remember to protect your clothes and/or use an old towel to prevent staining.

Makes 1 treatment

1 teaspoon ground turmeric
¼ cup coconut oil

1. Combine the turmeric and coconut oil in a small bowl. Mix well.

2. Apply to the scalp, massaging gently.

3. Allow the mixture to remain on the scalp for 30 minutes, then rinse thoroughly and shampoo.

4. Repeat once or twice per week until the dandruff is resolved.

HEARTBURN REMEDY Ⓖ

Is it any wonder that ginger is good for treating heartburn? I mean, really. Is it? We all know it settles a stomach, aids digestion, calms nausea, and is generally awesome for all things stomach-y. So, using it to treat heartburn should be a no-brainer, agreed? *Okay, fine,* I confess it seems kind of counterintuitive to me, too. Something along the lines of fighting fire with fire—adding hot and spicy ginger to an already burning situation—seems all wrong, but don't forget about its powerful anti-inflammatory properties! And don't forget how soothing ginger is to the stomach and intestines! And don't forget how it keeps food moving along in the digestive tract. And, ah, suddenly it all starts to make sense. The best way to relieve heartburn quickly is to chew on a piece of fresh ginger if you can stomach it (pardon the pun). If not, try this recipe for soothing ginger water. It takes all of a minute to make, maybe a minute and a half if you decide to sweeten it. In other words, relief is on the way!

Makes 1 treatment

One 1-inch knob fresh ginger, grated
1 cup chilled water
Raw honey (optional)

Combine all the ingredients in a glass. Stir to combine, then allow the ginger to settle. Add ice, if desired. Sip slowly.

STOMACH SOOTHER G T

We've all been there. Whether you went for the double bacon cheeseburger special or scarfed down *another* piece of birthday cake against your better judgment, you overdid it, and now you're going to have to pay. Your belly is rumbling, you're too full to move, and you've got that bloated, uncomfortable, why-did-I-do-that feeling. You *could* chew some chalky antacid tablets or maybe choke back a shot or two of that thick pink stuff, but wouldn't you rather go for something all natural that actually works and tastes good? Turmeric does wonders for a less-than-thrilled digestive system, thanks to its anti-inflammatory superpowers. It aids digestion and soothes an irritated digestive tract, so much so that research even suggests that the curcumin in turmeric may be an effective treatment in dealing with inflammatory bowel disorders. So, when you're full of nothing more than french fries and regret, restore happiness to your belly with this soothing and yummy elixir.

Makes 4 treatments

Juice of 2 lemons
¾ teaspoon ground turmeric
½ teaspoon fresh ginger, grated
2 tablespoons pure maple syrup
6 cups filtered water or sparkling water, if you prefer

Place all the ingredients in a small pitcher or mason jar. Shake or stir to combine. Serve over ice, if desired. Sip slowly.

THERAPEUTIC GINGER CHEWS FOR MORNING AND MOTION SICKNESS ⒢

I don't know where I got the notion, but before I had my first kid, I really, truly imagined I'd get pregnant and magically become this serene, rosy sort of earth mother, all shiny hair and glowing skin, with an effortlessly chic maternity wardrobe that flowed and flattered. It never crossed my mind that I'd spend 17 weeks with my first kid, then pretty much all nine months with the second, in a barftastic haze of nausea and exhaustion. (Not to mention that I'd be wearing maternity hand-me-downs from my sister-in-law who is literally about 9 inches taller than I am.) Glowing? Yeah, right.

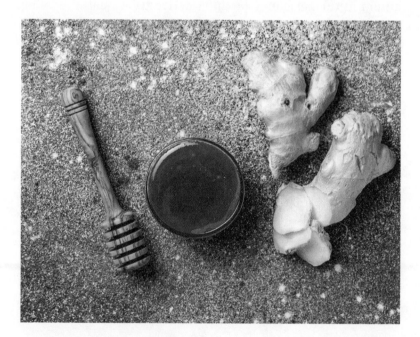

Of course, in the end it was all worth it, because I now have these two incredible little people whom I love more than I could ever have imagined was even possible. But that morning sickness—that was rough stuff: around-the-clock nausea, food aversions (I couldn't even *look* at broccoli), and, well, barfing. I tried all sorts of remedies, including straight lemon juice squeezed over crushed ice (a nightly "treat" my husband would make for me), motion sickness wristbands, and consuming my (steadily growing) body weight in frozen cheese ravioli. In the end, what I turned to most often were these sweet and spicy ginger chews—truly a medicinal miracle that are now a staple in our house, because they work so well for motion sickness, too. Ginger, of course, is a fantastic cure for upset stomachs and nausea, thanks to the compound [6]-gingerol that helps relax gastrointestinal muscles. This recipe is quite easy to make, though I do strongly recommend using a candy thermometer to be sure you get the texture just right. And speaking of candy, if you're looking for something that leans a little more toward the fun side, try the candied ginger on page 100—similar concept, but more of a treat than a treatment.

Makes 30 to 40 chews

Oil for pan
¼ cup packed shredded fresh ginger
2 cups water
¼ cup raw honey
¾ cup cane sugar

Continued

1. Lightly brush the bottom and sides of a small glass casserole dish or loaf pan with oil. Line with parchment, leaving a 2-inch overhang on the long sides; lightly brush the parchment with oil.

2. Combine the ginger and water in a medium saucepan over medium-low heat and simmer for 20 to 30 minutes, until the liquid has reduced by half. Strain the ginger, reserving 1 cup of the liquid.

3. Pour the ginger liquid into a large saucepan and add the honey and sugar; stir well. Insert a candy thermometer, then bring the mixture to a rolling boil over high heat, stirring until the sugar dissolves. Lower the heat to medium-high and cook, stirring occasionally, until the mixture reaches 260°F on the candy thermometer.

4. Immediately remove the pan from the heat and pour the mixture into the prepared dish. Allow the mixture to cool, uncovered, at room temperature, for at least 30 minutes and up to 1 day.

5. Lifting by the parchment overhang, remove the candy from the dish and transfer to a large cutting board. Using a sharp knife, cut into ¾-by-1¼-inch pieces; wrap each piece in waxed paper or cellophane.

ANTI-NAUSEA GINGER SYRUP Ⓖ

It seems ginger's uses when it comes to quelling nausea are just about endless. If ginger candy and ginger tea don't do it for you, there's always this incredibly simple syrup to stave off the queasies. You can stir it into sparkling water, add it to a mug of hot water, drizzle it over yogurt, or simply take it by the spoonful. With just a couple of common ingredients, it's a quick and easy way to find relief from nausea, motion sickness, indigestion, stomachaches, and the dreaded stomach flu. And, thanks to the raw honey, it's also antiviral, so it might even help as a preventive measure if you've been exposed to a stomach bug or another icky virus.

Makes about 2 cups syrup

½ cup ground ginger, or 1 cup fresh, peeled and chopped

2 cups water

1 cup raw honey

1. Combine the ginger and water in a medium saucepan over medium-low heat and simmer for 20 to 30 minutes, until the liquid has reduced by half.

2. Strain the liquid into a mason jar or other heatproof, lidded container. Discard the ginger solids or reserve for another use. Allow the liquid to cool until it's comfortable to handle, around 30 to 40 minutes, then stir in honey.

3. Store the syrup in the refrigerator for up to 3 months.

LONGEVITY TEA Ⓣ

In 2000, a *National Geographic* explorer and author named Dan Buettner rounded up a crew of anthropologists and other researchers to travel around the world and study communities with surprisingly high percentages of people living to age 100—what the world has come to know as Blue Zones. Among the big winners are Okinawa, Japan; Icaria, Greece; Ogliastra region, Sardinia; Loma Linda, California; and Nicoya Peninsula, Costa Rica. In all of the Blue Zones, not only do people tend to live longer, but they remain much healthier throughout their lives, experiencing less disease and greater happiness—fascinating, given the diversity in their diets, habits, and environments. In Okinawa, it seems, turmeric may be part of the answer to why the tiny island boasts one of the highest centenarian ratios in the world: about 6.5 in 10,000 people (versus 1.73 in 10,000 in the United States). Turmeric is one of the Okinawans' favorite spices, ever since they began importing it from India in the sixth century, and they drink tons of turmeric tea. Here, in this recipe, turmeric combines with jasmine tea (another important part of the Okinawan diet), resulting in a cup with a delicate earthiness and a relaxing, floral fragrance.

Makes 1 serving

1 teaspoon loose leaf jasmine tea

1 teaspoon ground turmeric, or 1 tablespoon grated fresh

Pinch of freshly ground black pepper

6 ounces boiling water

Sweetener such as raw honey, maple syrup, sugar, or whatever
you like, to taste

Combine the tea leaves, turmeric, and pepper in a nest strainer or infuser and place in a cup or mug. Pour the boiling water over the tea and let steep for 3 to 4 minutes. Sweeten as desired.

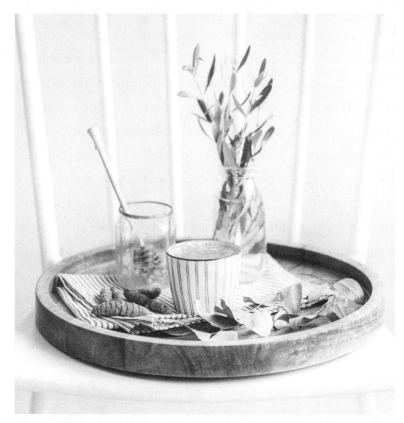

THE CURES-EVERYTHING GINGER BATH Ⓖ

Ginger is some pretty powerful stuff. Restorative, calming yet invigorating, and healing, it is so often the answer to what ails me. I want to boost my energy: ginger. I want to calm down: ginger. My stomach aches: ginger. My throat hurts: ginger. My skin itches: ginger. My muscles are sore: ginger. The warmth and mmm . . . that smell. I love it so much that sometimes I literally want to take a bath in it. And I have. This one, in fact. A hot bath filled with ginger (fresh or powdered) is an incredible way to detox, soothe sore muscles, and promote relaxation. *How?* Well, ginger contains compounds that are thought to stimulate circulation, warm the body, support digestion, and improve your metabolism. *Yeah, but how?* Well, for one thing, ginger in the bathwater will make you sweat. You'll sweat buckets. Rivers! That's part of the magic of ginger: it speeds up circulation, which in turn creates heat, which in turn—yep, you guessed it—makes you sweat. And all that sweating provides a clear path for toxins to get out of your bod. So, whether you want to alleviate cold and flu symptoms, undo a long night of questionable food and drink choices, soothe overworked muscles, or simply purge some of the nasty chemicals we're all exposed to every day, this bath is one of the best ways to get your detox on. Make sure to drink plenty of water before, during, and after the bath to replace the fluids because you're going to sweat. A lot. Even after you get out of the bath, you'll probably keep sweating for the next hour or so, so wear something light or just keep yourself wrapped in a towel. And if you have sensitive or allergy-prone skin, test ginger on a small patch of your skin for irritation before the bath.

Makes 1 treatment

½ cup grated fresh ginger

1. Fill a bathtub with hot water (as hot as you can safely stand it) and add the ginger. If you don't feel like having bits of ginger floating around while you soak, you can put the ginger in an old stocking or tie it up in some cheesecloth.

2. Get into the tub and soak for 20 to 30 minutes.

Note: If you have high blood pressure, diabetes, or a history of heart disease, don't use a ginger bath. If you're pregnant, have a liver condition, or are taking blood thinners, *consult with your doctor* before taking a bath in ginger. Ginger baths are not recommended for children under two years of age.

SLEEP-PROMOTING BATH SOAK Ⓖ

I once lived in a really quirky studio apartment. Not only was it small (the living area was just big enough for a bed or a couch, but not both, and my coffee table doubled as storage for my too-large shoe wardrobe), but curiously it had a fairly good-sized bathroom with a gorgeous, deep, step-up, art deco–style bathtub. The tub was square and built into the corner of the bathroom, which had a huge window and got tons of light. The thing was majestic and begged to be used for actual bath taking. And so, for a time, I got really into taking baths. As such, I developed a pretty serious bath salts (and bombs and oils . . .) habit that did quite a number on my wallet. So, after a while, in the name of frugality, I began to tinker with making my own bath products and came across this recipe that is supposed to be great for detoxifying the body. And it may do just that, which would make sense given that ginger produces a thermogenic effect (i.e., causes a slight increase in body temperature), helping you sweat out whatever shouldn't be in there. Epsom salts are said to "draw out" toxins, thanks to the power of magnesium and sulfate, but I find that they put me right to sleep every time I soak in them, so I categorize this stuff under "sleep promoting," which I think makes sense. This soothing treatment will help eliminate sleep-related woes from puffy eyes to cranky mornings, giving you plenty of zzzzs so you can look and feel your best.

Makes 1 treatment

⅓ cup Epsom salts

⅓ cup sea salt

⅓ cup baking soda

3 tablespoons ground ginger

1. Mix together all the ingredients and pour into a comfortably hot bath.

2. Try to soak for at least 20 minutes, then rinse off. Rehydrate with water before, during, and after the bath.

BEAUTY
SECRETS

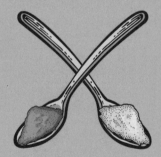

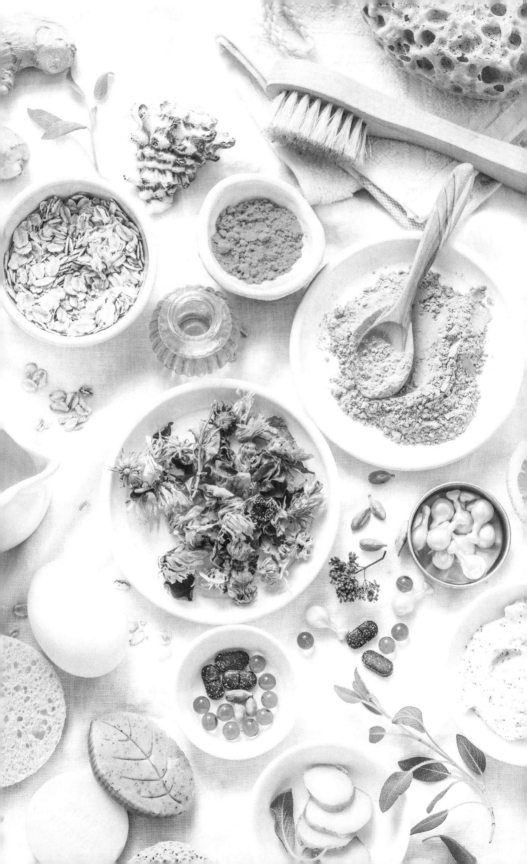

DIY BODY WRAP Ⓖ

If you've ever been to a fancy spa, you've seen body wraps on the list of services. In case you've wondered, as I did for ages, *what the heck is a body wrap?!* it's basically a full-body skin treatment. Like a mask. Except—and here's the funny part—you're then essentially rolled up in a fabric and/or plastic sheet like a human burrito. Ridiculous as that may seem (and it sort of *is*), the benefits are totally worth it. Lots of spas bill their wraps as a weight-loss hack. I have to confess to being a pretty major skeptic on that one (as if wrapping ourselves up like take-out orders from Chipotle was actually the secret!), but I do buy into the notion that it may reduce the appearance of cellulite and help tone the skin, especially when ginger enters the picture to rev up your circulation and draw out impurities. Here, as the body heats up under the wrap, the skin drinks in the ingredients, leaving it super soft, toned, and firm. If you are prone to dehydration or have had kidney dysfunction, you should skip the plastic wrap, but you can still enjoy the skin benefits of this treatment by simply using it as a body mask.

Makes 1 treatment

4 cups plain yogurt

2 cups raw honey

2 cups aloe vera gel

Two 4-inch pieces fresh ginger, grated

1. Mix together all the ingredients in a large bowl.

2. Line your bathtub with a towel, sheet, or soft (washable) blanket. Then, using your hands, spread the mask on your body and wrap each section with a piece of plastic wrap. Cover up, using the towel, sheet, or light blanket you've used to line the tub, and relax in the tub for 20 to 30 minutes.

3. Remove the cloth, remove the plastic wrap, rinse off the mask in the shower, and follow with a moisturizer.

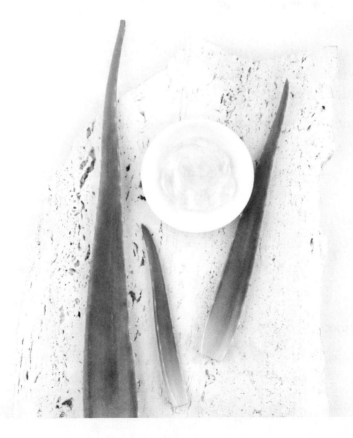

CRACKED HEEL REPAIR ⓣ

I've heard about people doing some crazy things in the name of soft, smooth feet, such as sleeping with lemons strapped to their heels and—get this—soaking their feet in tubs of warm water full of tiny fish called *Garra rufa* that exfoliate the skin by nibbling off dead skin cells. That's an *actual* spa treatment that people *pay* real money for! I kind of get it, though. Our feet go through a ton of wear and tear as we go about our lives, what with all that walking (especially in open-toed shoes), standing, exercising, and . . . merely existing. We're constantly putting stress on our feet, which is why they're prone to rebel on us from time to time in the form of flaking, peeling, calluses, and sometimes even *literally* cracking under the pressure. In addition to being unsightly, cracked heels can be incredibly painful and even dangerous, because they can become infected from bacteria, fungus, or a virus. The good news: This deeply hydrating and revitalizing foot treatment can alleviate symptoms and speed up the process of removing dead skin cells. The curcumin in turmeric increases the production of new blood vessels and connective tissue and helps replace old, craggy skin, protecting your heels from further damage. So, without further ado . . .

Makes 1 treatment

½ teaspoon ground turmeric

2 teaspoons coconut oil

1. Soak your feet in warm water for 10 to 15 minutes to soften the skin.

2. After soaking your feet, use a pumice stone or foot file to scrub the heels, removing dead skin cells and smoothing out the area.

3. Combine the turmeric and coconut oil in a small bowl. Mix well, then apply the mixture to your heels, gently massaging it into the skin. Leave the treatment on for 10 to 15 minutes, then wash your feet with warm water and mild soap. Pat dry. Repeat daily.

Note: If you have chronically dry or cracked heels that don't respond to self-care, talk to your health-care provider to rule out certain health problems, such as skin conditions, thyroid issues, vitamin deficiency, or weight issues, that could be causing your cracked heels.

GINGER AND MUSTARD FOOT SOAK Ⓖ

If the idea of mustard on your feet instead of, say, on a hot dog has you scratching your head, know this: mustard baths have been around for a long time, particularly in England, where they've been used forever as a remedy for colds and more. As far back as ancient Rome, people were soaking in mustard for its detoxifying benefits as well as its power to help with stress, sleeplessness, muscle aches, chills, and general fatigue. The one-two punch of ginger and mustard works particularly well as a foot bath because it not only rejuvenates tired feet, it helps relax the mind and detoxify the system straight through the soles. Both mustard and ginger stimulate sweat glands and increase circulation in the body, which helps draw out impurities and toxins. Because your whole being is connected to your feet, taking good care of them, including making this footbath part of your regular routine, does wonders for your overall health. Follow with a thick slathering of rich lotion or a luxurious balm, pull on a cozy pair of socks, and—look at that—you're a new person.

Makes 1 treatment

1½ tablespoons dry mustard
2 tablespoons peeled and grated fresh ginger

Combine the mustard and ginger in a footbath or basin large enough to accommodate your feet. Add enough warm (not hot) water to cover your feet. Relax and soak your feet for 15 to 20 minutes.

TURMERIC BODY SCRUB Ⓣ

I always used to think that the only reason to use a body scrub was to, you know, scrub your skin smooth, but it turns out that there's more to the story than mere exfoliation. When you use a body scrub, you're not just giving your skin a buff for texture's sake; you're also taking in vitamins, minerals, and other nutrients that benefit your body in a variety of ways. *Who knew?* The coffee in this invigorating scrub helps with fluid buildup, because caffeine tones and tightens the skin and, according to research, may also reduce the appearance of cellulite. Plus, coffee is full of antioxidants, which nourish your skin, fight the signs of aging, and may also help release toxins. Sugar, with its natural glycolic acid, helps remove dead skin and acts as a natural humectant, while coconut oil adds vitamin E, essential amino acids, and lauric acid in addition to luxurious moisture. Of course, turmeric also adds extra antioxidant and anti-inflammatory firepower to the mix and helps brighten and even out your skin tone. In other words, if you're looking for fresh, glowing, smooth, and moisturized skin, then you came to the right place. If, on the other hand, you happen to like your cellulite and dull skin, you should definitely skip this scrub. Definitely.

Makes about 2 cups scrub

Continued

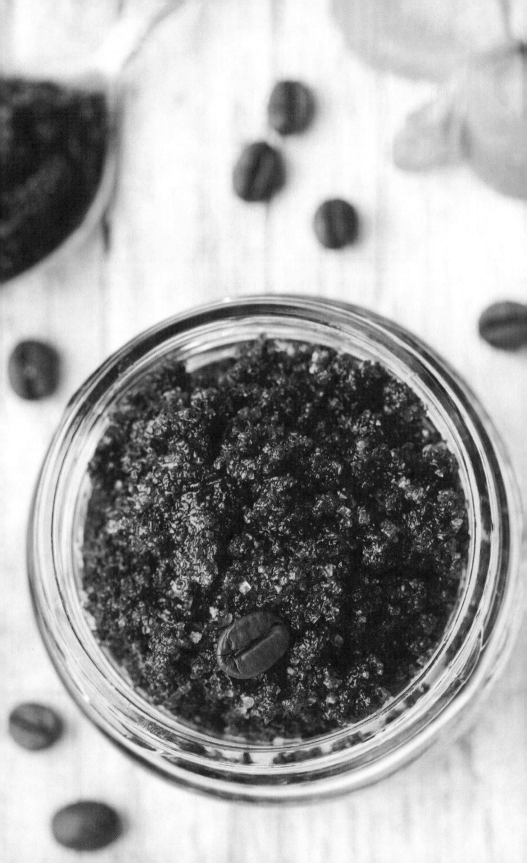

½ cup coconut oil, melted and cooled slightly

1 cup ground coffee (preferably organic, unflavored)

1 cup sugar

1 teaspoon ground turmeric

1. Combine the melted coconut oil and coffee grounds in a small bowl. Stir to thoroughly mix the ingredients and set the bowl aside.

2. Combine the sugar and turmeric in a medium bowl. Stir them together to fully mix and get rid of any chunks.

3. Pour the oil mixture into the sugar. Use your hands or a spatula to thoroughly mix.

4. Transfer the mixture into a jar or other container with a tight-fitting lid.

5. To use, apply to wet skin, scrub in circular motions, and rinse off. Be sure to use this with hot water to help the coconut oil move through your pipes so that it doesn't clog up your drain.

Note: Much as I love to repurpose all kinds of kitchen waste, you're better off not using spent coffee grounds here. Coffee that hasn't been previously brewed will be much more potent than used grounds.

GINGER BODY SCRUB Ⓖ

If I hadn't been the one to write this book and saw it on a bookstore shelf, I would probably have picked it up, flipped directly to the index, and looked to see whether (please please please) there was a DIY version of my most favorite body scrub on earth—one I bought at a fancy cosmetics store for years. It is one of the best-smelling, happy-inducing, calming-yet-invigorating products around. Lucky for us both, I *am* the one to write this book, so here is a pretty freaking fantastic scrub that I now make myself instead of shelling out for the fancy store-bought version. You're welcome! With the intoxicating scent of ginger and the combination of sugar, salt, and olive oil, this scrub will leave your skin silky smooth, moisturized, and refreshed. And it doesn't cost $20 a tub. Bonus!

Makes about 1½ cups scrub

One 3-inch piece fresh ginger, chopped roughly

1½ cups sugar

2 tablespoons olive oil

½ cup very fine sea salt

Juice of ½ lime

1 tablespoon liquid castile soap

1. Combine the ginger, ½ cup of the sugar, and the olive oil in a food processor or high-speed blender. Process until very smooth.

2. Transfer the mixture to a bowl and add the remaining sugar and other ingredients. Stir to combine.

3. Store in an airtight container.

4. To use: Apply to wet skin. Scrub in a circular motion. Rinse.

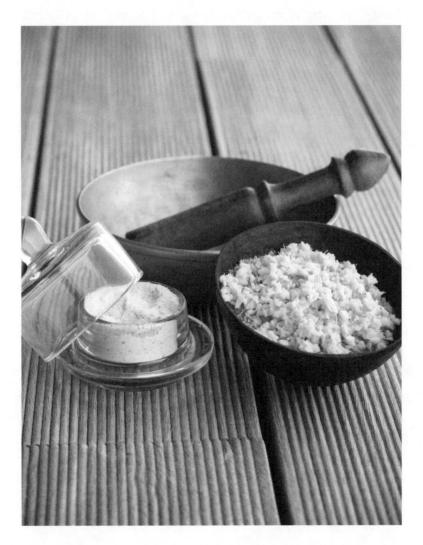

WARMING MASSAGE OIL Ⓖ

This anti-inflammatory, pain-relieving, yummy-smelling, all-around-soothing balm really couldn't be simpler to make. With just two ingredients—ginger and oil—it's a lifesaver for anyone suffering from aches, pains, tension, sore muscles and joints, arthritis, nerve pain, or even menstrual cramps. Gently massage it (or have a loved one lend a hand) into wherever you need it and enjoy luxurious, warm relief. If you want to get fancy, you can add several drops of eucalyptus, peppermint, or camphor oil to the finished product, all of which add a cooling sensation to the oil and further help it boost circulation. To kick up the pain relief yet another notch, consider adding ½ teaspoon or so of cayenne pepper to the mixture. *I know!* But, see, the funny thing is that cayenne contains a compound called capsaicin, which is a natural pain reliever. When it's applied to the skin, your brain thinks it's been exposed to extreme heat, which sends your pain-blocking neurotransmitters into high gear. Pretty cool . . . *er* hot, actually. I especially like to use the oil straight up, without any of those add-ins, on my feet as part of an at-home pedicure. It's divine. Before you get started with ginger oil, be sure to do a test on a small area of skin, and don't use it on broken or irritated skin.

Makes about 1½ cups massage oil

1 cup shredded fresh ginger

1½ cups olive, sesame, or almond oil

1. Preheat the oven to 150°F.

2. Combine the ginger and oil in an ovenproof bowl or casserole dish and place it in the oven. Heat for 2 hours to
   infuse.

3. Remove from the oven and strain the oil through a
   cheesecloth-lined funnel into a clean bottle or jar. Allow to
   cool completely, then seal with a lid.

4. Store the oil in a cool, dark place for up to 6 months.

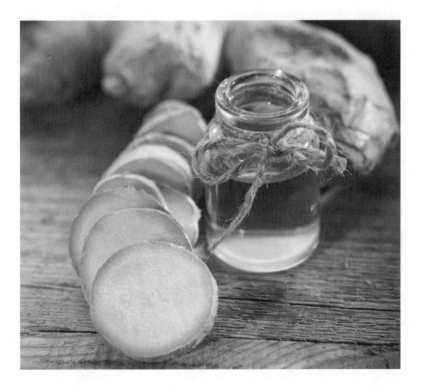

CHOCOLATE-GINGER BATH Ⓖ

If you've ever dreamed of taking a bath in chocolate, here's your shot! This soothing soak, made with ingredients that not only smell amazing but also have some pretty incredible benefits for your skin, is sort of an East-meets-West or—more exactly—a Willy-Wonka-meets-the-spa-at-the-Mandarin-Oriental kind of sensory experience. With an indulgent combination of ingredients that soften, smooth, detoxify, invigorate, and tone the skin, this is a fabulous recipe to make in bulk for gift giving and/or to keep on hand in case you're hit with a sudden chocolate emergency. For maximum cuteness, package the salts in little glass milk bottles—it'll look like chocolate milk.

Makes about 5 cups salts

1 cup Epsom salts
1 cup coarse sea salt
¼ cup unsweetened cocoa powder
2 tablespoons ground ginger
2 cups powdered milk
½ cup cornstarch
½ cup baking soda

1. Combine the Epsom salts, sea salt, cocoa powder, and ginger in a medium bowl. Mix well. Set aside.

2. Mix together the powdered milk, cornstarch, and baking soda in a separate bowl.

3. Layer the ginger mixture and the milk mixture into glass jar(s), cellophane bags, or those adorable little milk bottles.

4. To use: Add ½ cup to warm bath water. Swirl it around the water to mix it in. Relax and enjoy.

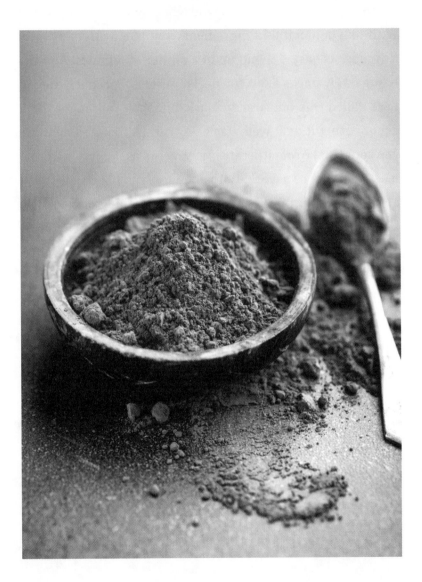

RADIANCE-BOOSTING FACIAL MASK G T

Want an easy, DIY ginger face mask that'll leave your skin feeling clean, moisturized, and downright glowing?! Yeah, you do! With only a handful of ingredients you likely already stock, this mask is easy to whip up in a matter of minutes. And the best part? It smells like a cookie. I'm serious. I probably should have called this Gingersnap Mask, but then you might think about eating it and, well, don't do that. (Although I suppose you could . . .) Aromatherapeutic benefits aside, this is a great mask to use once a week. With an ingredient list that is full of antioxidants, anti-inflammatories, and soothing humectants, this stuff stimulates blood flow (there's that glow), helps draw toxins from the pores, exfoliates the skin's surface, and generally tightens and brightens everything up. Plus it's suitable for all skin types. Be sure to use it the same day you make it to prevent any icky bacteria from growing. Growing and glowing— much more than a one-letter difference.

Makes 1 treatment

1 teaspoon raw honey

1 tablespoon plain Greek yogurt

1 tablespoon grated fresh ginger

¼ teaspoon sea salt

¼ teaspoon unsweetened cocoa powder

¼ teaspoon ground turmeric

¼ teaspoon ground nutmeg

¼ teaspoon ground cinnamon

¼ teaspoon ground cloves

Combine all the ingredients in a small bowl. Spread the mixture onto your face and let it sit for 10 to 15 minutes, then rinse off. Pat dry and follow with your usual moisturizer.

ACNE-FIGHTING TURMERIC MASK T

I love any product that can multitask, in or out of the kitchen, and when it comes to skin care, well . . . you want a product that simultaneously fights breakouts, wrinkles, acne scars, and oily skin, all in one fell swoop. This turmeric mask is just that—a skin care wizard that is gentle, full of natural ingredients, and most important, effective against acne. With an ingredient list that sounds more like a delicious dressing than a skin care treatment (note to self: turmeric, lemon, and yogurt dressing in next book), this stuff is an antioxidant and anti-inflammatory wonderland that's ideal for anyone, really, but especially those dealing with acne, as it calms inflammation, kills microorganisms on the skin, and helps fade dark spots. While *all* of the ingredients in the mask contain antioxidants, yogurt also brings the addition of probiotics to the table, raw honey is naturally antibacterial, and turmeric—of course—takes care of cell damage, inflammation, and dull skin. Use this stuff regularly and you'll definitely see clearer, brighter skin!

Makes 1 or 2 treatments

¼ cup plain yogurt

1 tablespoon raw honey

½ teaspoon ground turmeric

½ teaspoon fresh lemon juice

1. Mix together all the ingredients in a small bowl until thoroughly combined.

2. Apply the mask to your face, being careful to avoid your eyes, and leave it on your skin for 15 to 20 minutes.

3. Rinse with lukewarm water, pat dry, and moisturize as usual. Repeat once or twice a week.

4. Any leftover mask can be stored in the refrigerator for up to 3 days.

Note: To remove any lingering yellow tint on the skin, simply give it a swipe of witch hazel or your go-to toner on a cotton ball.

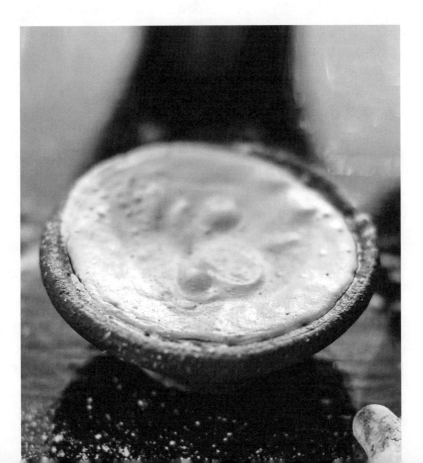

PURIFYING FACIAL MASK Ⓖ Ⓣ

For all the time you spend focused on cleansing your skin, isn't it funny how one of the most surefire ways to get a clear, glowing complexion is to smear dirt all over your face? Well, kind of. Clay and charcoal (both dirt at the end of the day; see what I'm saying?) are powerful skin purifiers—mainstays, in fact, on the treatment menus at most high-end spas. Why? Because they pull toxins, bacteria, dead skin cells, and oil from your pores in a heartbeat. Pair those bad girls with inflammation-reducing turmeric, circulation-boosting ginger, and moisturizing honey, and you're looking at one foolproof way to get positively radiant skin. If, by chance, you have a particularly fair complexion and end up with slightly yellow skin after removing the mask, *do not panic*. Simply give your skin a swipe of witch hazel or your go-to toner on a cotton ball, and I promise you'll stop looking like one of the Simpsons.

Makes 1 treatment

1 teaspoon charcoal powder

½ teaspoon bentonite clay

1 teaspoon ground turmeric

1 teaspoon raw honey

½ teaspoon ground ginger

1. Combine all the ingredients in a bowl. Add enough water to form a paste.

3. Massage onto your skin and leave on for 10 minutes.

4. Rinse with warm water. Pat dry.

5. Follow with your favorite moisturizer.

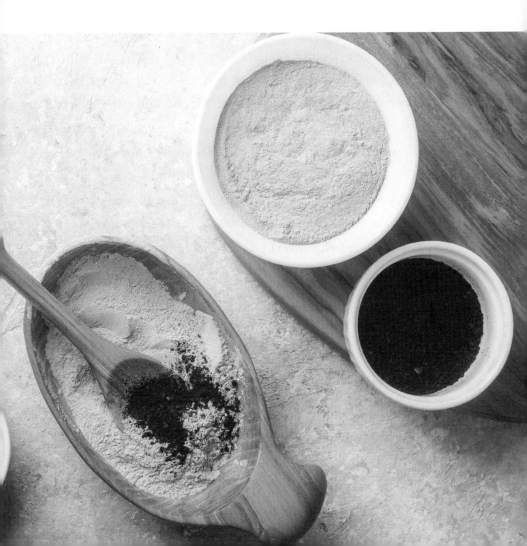

WRINKLE-REDUCING
EYE TREATMENT Ⓖ

When I look in the mirror, I mostly see the same face that's been staring back at me for my whole life. Somehow, it's hard to see age on our own countenance. Except for those times when we look in the mirror and that's *all* we see! I've noticed more lines around my eyes, more furrow in my brow, more sag here and there. And I know it's inevitable and that there's something to be said for aging gracefully and being comfortable in our own skin. I try to remember that they're called laugh lines for a reason, and some of that "aging" around my eyes is just evidence of a life well lived. But is there really any harm in *trying* to turn back time a little? I think not. When it comes to protecting skin cells from the free radicals that cause fine lines and wrinkles, ginger comes to play: it contains about 40 antioxidants, including vitamin C, curcumin, and farnesol, all of which bring antiaging benefits to skin. When applied directly to the skin around the eyes, it stimulates circulation, bringing a rush of blood to just the right spot. Combined with moisturizing and rejuvenating honey, this treatment is a powerful potion to keep you looking fresh and bright eyed. Just, for goodness' sake, please use care when applying the treatment, because if you get this stuff in your eyes, it will B-U-R-N.

Makes 1 treatment

1 teaspoon ginger juice (store-bought or squeezed from
  several tablespoons of grated fresh ginger)

1 teaspoon raw honey

1. Combine the ginger and honey in a small bowl. Mix well.

2. Gently massage the mixture into the skin under your eyes,
   taking great care not to get it in your eyes. Allow the treatment to sit on the skin for 1 hour.

3. Gently remove the mixture with lukewarm water. Pat dry
   and follow with an eye cream.

ANTI-INFLAMMATORY AND EXFOLIATING FACE POWDER Ⓣ

As most people who don't reside under a rock are well aware, exfoliating is a must for beautiful, healthy skin. And while it's quite tempting to load up on fancy, beautifully packaged, promise-laden skin-perfecting products, such as peels, exfoliating wipes, glycolic serums, and rejuvenating masks, there's a super minimalist and unbelievably effective approach to skin care that will renew the heck out of your skin: dry cleansing powders. Sometimes called cleansing grains, powdered facial cleansers are a versatile three-in-one skin care wonder (the three are: cleanser, exfoliator, and mask, in case that wasn't clear) made from stuff like ground oats, herbs, nuts, clay, or other nourishing ingredients that, when combined with a bit of water in the palm of your hand, will cleanse and exfoliate your face in a flash. Here, oatmeal and almond meal gently exfoliate and moisturize, while turmeric soothes, brightens, calms irritation, and helps to give dull skin a pretty glow. My favorite thing about this stuff, however, is that—because it's dry—it'll keep forever, so if you've got the bathroom real estate, you can make a really huge batch and keep it around for a good long time.

Makes about 1 cup face powder

½ cup rolled oats

3 tablespoons almond meal (a.k.a. almond flour)

1 teaspoon ground turmeric

OPTIONAL ADDITIONS:

1 to 2 tablespoons chamomile flowers, for sensitive skin

10 to 15 drops essential oils, such as lavender, tea tree, or rose

1. Place all the ingredients in a food processor or clean coffee grinder and process until you achieve a fine powder.

2. To use as a daily cleanser: Put a teaspoon or two into the palm of your hand and add enough water to form a paste. Use as you would any cleanser. Rinse thoroughly and follow with your usual beauty routine.

3. To use as a mask: Place a teaspoon or two of the powder into the palm of your hand and add enough water, plain yogurt (for extra brightening and nourishment), or coconut oil (for a moisturizing boost) to form a thick but spreadable paste. Apply it to your face, being careful to avoid your eyes. Leave for 10 to 15 minutes, then rinse with lukewarm water, pat dry, and moisturize as usual. Repeat once or twice a week.

INVIGORATING FACIAL SCRUB G

If you make the mistake, as I have, of perusing the Internet to find out how often you should use a face scrub, here's what it will tell you: Exfoliating daily is a *must* for perfect skin. Wait—no—daily exfoliating is way, *way* too harsh on your skin. Do it less often. Do it twice a week. No, twice a month. And use a chemical exfoliator. No, use a granular one. Aaaaaahhhhh! Why so hard? You'd think I'd looked up, "What is the meaning of life?" After digging my way out of the virtual skin-exfoliating rabbit hole, I came to my own conclusion, which is that different skin responds to different beauty routines, and you kind of have to know your skin to know what's right. Duh. I use a scrub as often as I remember to, which works out to about twice a week. This is the one I use most often. With cleansing and brightening lemon, moisturizing coconut oil, gently exfoliating baking soda, and—of course—antiaging and antioxidant ginger, this all-natural scrub will have you looking and feeling like a million bucks.

Makes about 1½ cups scrub

1 cup sugar or baking soda

½ cup coconut oil or olive oil

1 teaspoon grated fresh ginger

1 teaspoon grated lemon zest

1 or 2 drops ginger oil and/or lemon oil (optional)

1. Place all the ingredients in a small bowl. Mix well to combine.

2. Transfer into an airtight container. Store the scrub in the refrigerator in its container for up to 2 weeks.

3. To use: Wash your face with your usual cleanser. Apply a small amount of the scrub to wet skin and massage gently in a circular motion, being careful to avoid the eye area. Rinse well and pat dry. Follow with a moisturizer.

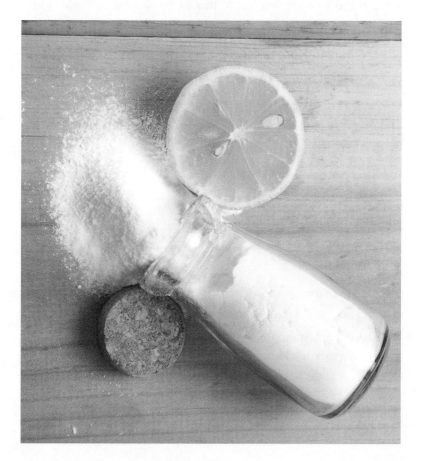

PUMPKIN AND TURMERIC FADE TREATMENT FOR SKIN SPOTS Ⓣ

Whatcha got there—age spots? Sun spots? Acne scars? Chicken pox marks? While there may be more than one reason for the marks on your skin, here's a surefire way to naturally and comfortably go after them. Like peels and laser treatments that lighten dark spots, turmeric has been shown to treat, fade, and correct the appearance of sun damage and other types of hyperpigmentation on the skin, but without the cost and side effects. Here, pumpkin (an excellent source of zinc, alphahydroxy acids, and vitamins A and C to give skin a radiant glow and even the complexion), honey (to brighten and soften your skin), and turmeric (in this case a skin-lightening genius) work together to resurface and revitalize your skin, giving you a softer, healthier, and more even complexion. You can kiss that spotty situation goodbye!

Makes 1 treatment

1 tablespoon pumpkin puree

½ teaspoon ground turmeric

1 teaspoon raw honey, warmed for a few seconds in a microwave so it is pourable

1. Combine all the ingredients in a small bowl and mix well.

2. Apply the mixture to the affected area (face, neck, chest, or back) with your fingers or a small brush.

3. Leave on for 10 to 15 minutes, then rinse with lukewarm water. To remove any lingering yellow tint on the skin, simply give it a swipe of witch hazel or your go-to toner on a cotton ball, then pat dry and follow with a moisturizer.

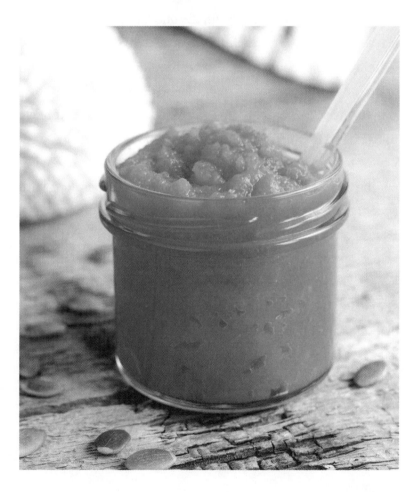

HOMEMADE WHITENING TOOTHPASTE ⓣ

One indisputable fact about turmeric is that it stains like hell. It'll stain your clothes, your skin, your counters, and . . . your toothbrush. Yes, your *toothbrush*! Wondering why and how turmeric would ever end up on your toothbrush in the first place? Well, if you brushed your teeth with it, you'd end up with turmeric on your toothbrush. As it turns out, the one place turmeric doesn't leave stains is on your teeth. Truth. In fact, it is a pretty fantastic whitening product, thanks to tetrahydrocurcumin, a compound in turmeric that accounts for its lightening properties. Yep, turmeric and coconut oil—probably two of the least likely things you'd instinctively grab when thinking about how to get whiter teeth—can subtly and gently brighten your smile without the chemicals and tooth sensitivity that often tag along with over-the-counter whitening strips or whitening toothpaste. Using a turmeric-based whitening paste a few times a week can help keep stains from coffee, wine, and the like at bay, but don't expect a blindingly white outcome. Think: Subtle. Think: Understated. Because I like a minty-fresh toothpaste, I add a few drops of food-grade peppermint oil to my homemade concoction. This is an optional step, but one I highly recommend. One final tip: Don't use your fancy electric toothbrush with this stuff. I'm not sure I've mentioned it, but, um, turmeric stains—it'll stain your fancy brush. Use a cheap one that you can throw away when the bright yellow bristles start to really freak you out.

Makes about ½ cup toothpaste

¼ cup coconut oil

2 tablespoons ground turmeric

2 tablespoons baking soda

5 to 10 drops food-grade peppermint oil (optional)

1. Place all the ingredients in a small bowl and stir well to thoroughly combine. Transfer the mixture to a small mason jar or—my favorite—a squeezable silicone travel tube.

2. To use, squeeze a small amount of toothpaste onto your toothbrush or, using a small spoon or popsicle stick, remove a pea-sized amount from the jar and spread it on your toothbrush. Brush as you would with any toothpaste for about 2 minutes. Rinse and spit. For best results, repeat once or twice a week.

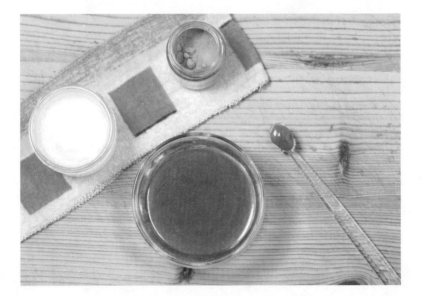

LIP PLUMPER Ⓖ

Maybe you weren't born with Angelina's pout. Or Kylie's. (Or Daffy Duck's?) Or maybe your lips have lost some of their oomph as you've aged. Whatever the case may be, getting plump, voluptuous lips that are smooth, soft, and downright kissable is as easy as grabbing a knob of fresh ginger. Well, almost. Just like many of the expensive beauty store products, this DIY plumper relies on spicy ginger, cinnamon, and cayenne—mild (yet safe) irritants—to increase blood circulation in the lip area so that they look puffier. No visits to the dermatologist or needles required! For the perfect pout, use a good lip scrub to remove flakes, moisturize with a hydrating lip balm, then give this tingly DIY plumper a try. Now, pucker up!

Makes about 1 tablespoon plumper

1 tablespoon coconut oil

1 teaspoon olive oil

¼ teaspoon cinnamon essential oil

½ teaspoon ground ginger, or ¼ teaspoon ginger essential oil

¼ teaspoon cayenne pepper

1. Melt the coconut oil in a small bowl by placing it in a microwave on HIGH for 15 seconds at a time. Add the remaining ingredients and stir to combine. Set aside to cool.

2. Once cooled, apply a few drops of the lip plumper to your lips, lightly massaging it in a circular motion. Leave it on for 5 to 10 minutes, and then rinse with cool water or leave it on for a lasting effect. Store any remaining lip plumper at room temperature in a small, airtight container.

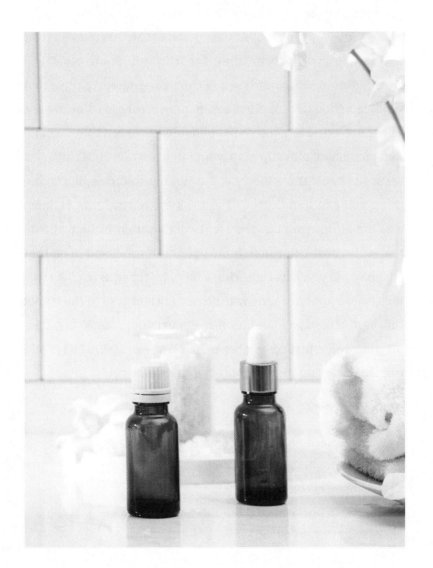

TINTED MOISTURIZER Ⓖ Ⓣ

Sometimes DIYing is almost comically easy. Such as when, for example, you throw a few household ingredients into a spray bottle and call it an all-purpose cleaner, which I do often and you can, too! (See *The Apple Cider Vinegar Companion* and *The Baking Soda Companion*.) At the far end of the spectrum is stuff like building furniture, tiling a bathroom, doing electrical work, spinning yarn, and raising chickens—undertakings that require a good deal of precision, patience, time, and/or money. These are areas in which I do not dabble. So, even though making homemade makeup may sound like next-level DIYing, rest assured that if it's something I'm willing to tackle, it's something you can handle, too. The trickiest part of this makeup making is figuring out the right combination of ingredients to get the best color match for your skin tone, and even that isn't hard so much as requiring a bit of trial and error. The turmeric here not only adds warmth and brightness to the tint of this light-coverage foundation, it's nourishing, too. When mixing your color, just remember to go slow—you can always add more of a certain ingredient to get the shade you're after.

Makes about ½ cup

3 tablespoons almond oil, coconut oil, or jojoba oil

2 tablespoons shea butter

1 tablespoon cocoa butter

1 tablespoon beeswax pellets

⅛ teaspoon vitamin E oil

1 tablespoon zinc oxide powder (optional, for sun protection), cornstarch, or arrowroot powder

¼ to ½ teaspoon unsweetened cocoa powder

¼ to ½ teaspoon ground nutmeg

⅛ to ¼ teaspoon ground turmeric

1 pinch to ¼ teaspoon ground cloves

1 pinch to ¼ teaspoon ground ginger

1 pinch to ¼ teaspoon ground sage (optional; helps correct redness)

1. Place the almond oil, shea butter, cocoa butter, beeswax, and vitamin E oil in a heatproof bowl set over a pot of simmering water and melt, stirring occasionally. Remove from the heat and allow to cool slightly.

2. Whisk in the zinc oxide (if using) or the cornstarch, then start mixing in your pigments, testing the mixture occasionally on your wrist to get a good color match. Start with the smallest quantity of suggested ingredient and add more as needed.

3. Pour into a small metal tin, mason jar, or a handy-dandy squeezable silicone travel tube and allow to cool.

4. Apply the makeup with your fingers or a sponge. Set with powder, if desired.

HOMEMADE BRONZER ⓣ

This is one of my most favorite beauty hacks of all time—mostly because it's so easy, it's almost stupid. It is literally as simple as starting to mix together the dry ingredients for a cookie recipe. And if you were making cookies and combined these same four or five ingredients, you'd only be halfway through making the dough. So, you see, making your own bronzer is way easier than making cookies, and making cookies can be pretty freaking easy. Other reasons to make your own bronzer? It's weird-ingredient-free, incredibly inexpensive, and a safe way to get a sun-kissed look without actually having to spend any time in the sun (a.k.a. UVA ray–free). So, even in the dead of winter you can get that bright, fresh, just-stepped-off-the-beach glow that only a good bronzer can deliver. As we're all different, you'll have to play around with the proportions a bit to get a shade that's just right for your skin tone. The measurements below are a rough guide to get you started. Just keep this in mind: Cinnamon = glow. Cocoa = tan. Nutmeg = sun-kissed. Turmeric = brightness and warmth.

Makes a small jar of loose powder

1 tablespoon ground cinnamon

1 teaspoon unsweetened cocoa powder

1 teaspoon ground nutmeg

¼ to ½ teaspoon ground turmeric

2 teaspoons cornstarch or arrowroot powder

1. Mix together all the ingredients—proportions adjusted to complement your skin tone—in a small bowl, breaking up any clumps until smooth. Pass the mixture through a fine-mesh sieve a few times to ensure a perfectly smooth consistency. If necessary, use a mortar and pestle or a coffee or spice grinder to achieve a finer powder. That's it!

2. Store in a small jar or empty bronzer container that's been cleaned out.

3. To use: Dip a big makeup brush into your bronzer and lightly dust the areas where the sun would naturally hit your face (cheeks, nose, chin, forehead, etc.).

Note: The above recipe is for a loose powder. To use in a makeup compact, add 10 to 15 drops of essential oil to the bronzer when mixing your ingredients together, then pack into a clean compact. Using the back of a spoon works well to tamp down the powder.

GOLDEN TURMERIC EYE SHADOW ⓣ

When I was a kid, I had a friend whose dad was a microbiologist for a major consumer goods company. Their medicine cabinet was a health and beauty wonderland: instead of nail polish remover, they had pure acetone (the active ingredient in most commercial nail polish removers); they had bottles and jars of all kinds of powders, lotions, and unidentifiable goop that had come home from the lab for their family's personal use. To a couple of eight-year-old girls who'd lost interest in Barbies, this meant hours of entertainment, mixing up oozing, bubbling "potions" in the bathroom, which we'd occasionally try to sell door-to-door around the neighborhood. (I recall getting into trouble for hocking our wares and having to make the rounds, giving money back to kind older neighbors who'd bought our snake oil.) So, given my history, it's really no surprise that I've managed to make a career out of mixing stuff up—that's cooking, after all. Beyond food, I do still get a thrill out of concocting magic potions in the bathroom, which probably accounts for 80 percent of my motivation to DIY personal care products, such as this amazing DIY eye shadow. Sure, making your own makeup and other beauty products is safer, all natural, better for the environment, better for your body, better for your wallet, yada yada yada, but let's not lose sight of the fact that

Continued

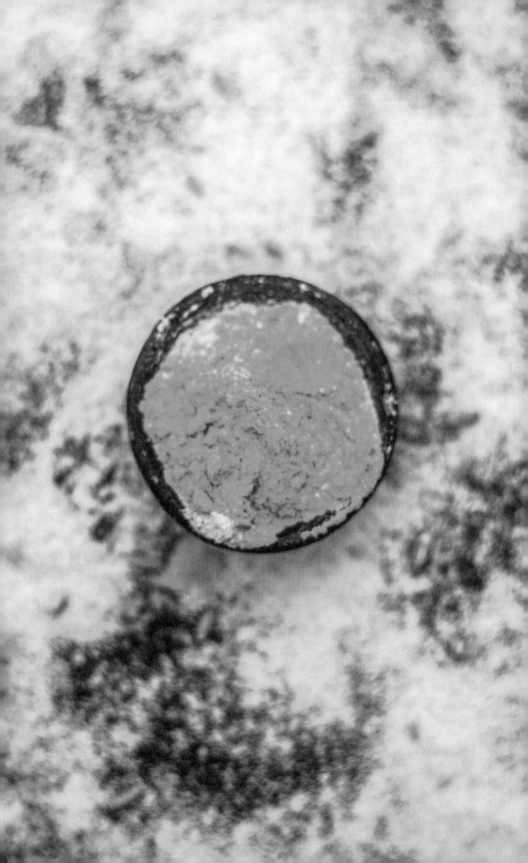

it is also *crazy fun* to do! This golden eye shadow is easy to mix together, flattering on just about any skin tone, and easily customizable to suit your color and shimmer preferences. Just don't try selling it door-to-door. My mom will make you give the money back.

Makes about 1 teaspoon eye shadow

¼ to ½ teaspoon arrowroot powder or cornstarch

¼ teaspoon shea butter

1 pinch to ⅛ teaspoon ground turmeric

1 pinch to ⅛ teaspoon cacao powder, unsweetened cocoa powder, or ground nutmeg

Sprinkle of mica powder (optional, for shimmer)

1. Mix all the ingredients—proportions adjusted to complement your skin tone—in a small bowl, breaking up any clumps until smooth. Pass the mixture through a fine-mesh sieve a few times to ensure a perfectly smooth consistency.

2. To use: Dip your fingertip or a small brush into the eye shadow. Tap off any excess and gently swipe across your eyelid as you would any other eye shadow.

3. Remove as you would any other eye shadow, using your favorite makeup remover or good old-fashioned soap and water.

SPLIT ENDS TREATMENT Ⓖ

I think we can probably agree that few things feel as good as a good hair day. And a bad hair day? Oh my! Pity the fools who cross us on those days! Some hair woes, such as a bad cut or a botched color job, just need time (and perhaps a flattering hat), but when it comes to one of the most common hair troubles—split ends—ginger can really come to the rescue. It penetrates, moisturizes, and—thanks to a plethora of vitamins, minerals, and fatty acids—actually strengthens your hair, sealing those mood-ruining split ends that dare to show up between salon appointments. When your hair is extra-parched, as is the case when you have split ends, this deep-conditioning mask is an absolute godsend.

Makes 1 treatment

1 tablespoon jojoba oil
1 tablespoon grated fresh ginger

1. Combine the oil and ginger in a small bowl. Massage the mixture into your hair, concentrating on the ends. Put on a plastic shower cap or wrap your hair in a towel, if desired.

2. After 30 minutes, rinse and shampoo as usual.

HAIR GROWTH TREATMENT Ⓖ

Maybe you chopped your hair into a trendy little bob and now you're pining for those long, cascading tresses of yore. Or perhaps you're experiencing that truly unsettling (though normal) postpartum hair loss. Whatever the reason, you want your hair to grow. Like, yesterday. Well, there's good news and bad news. The bad news is that you're going to have to be patient. Even with all its near-magical powers, ginger can't make your hair grow overnight. But it *can* provide your scalp with some serious TLC, which will set you well on your way to long and luxurious locks. So, whether you're growing out your bangs or have your eye on some sort of crazy Pinterest braid situation, use this treatment once or twice a month to increase blood flow and bring added nourishment and oxygen to your scalp and hair follicles.

Makes 1 treatment

¼ teaspoon grated fresh ginger
2 tablespoons olive oil

1. Combine the oil and ginger in a small saucepan. Cook gently for about 5 minutes over medium heat until the ginger just begins to brown. Remove from the heat and allow it to cool. Strain out and discard the ginger solids, reserving the oil.

2. Apply to the scalp and leave on for 5 to 10 minutes, then rinse thoroughly. Follow with shampoo and conditioner.

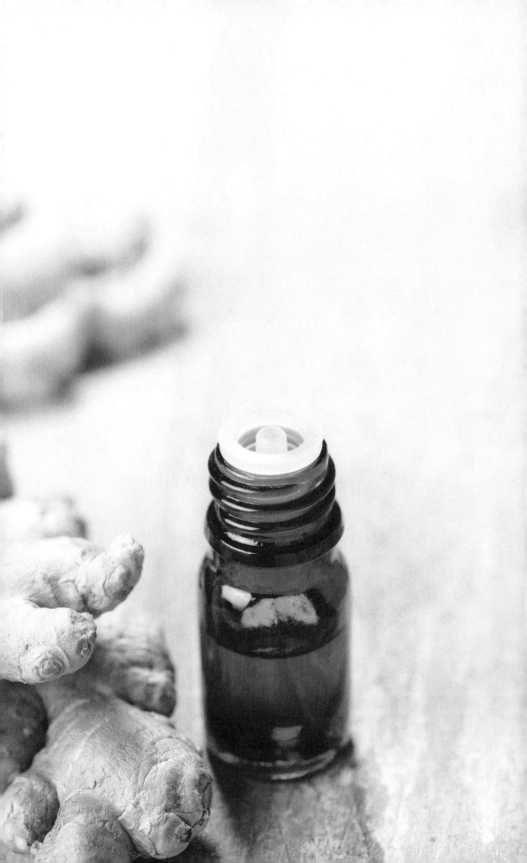

AROUND
THE HOME

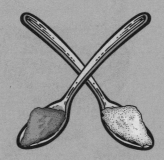

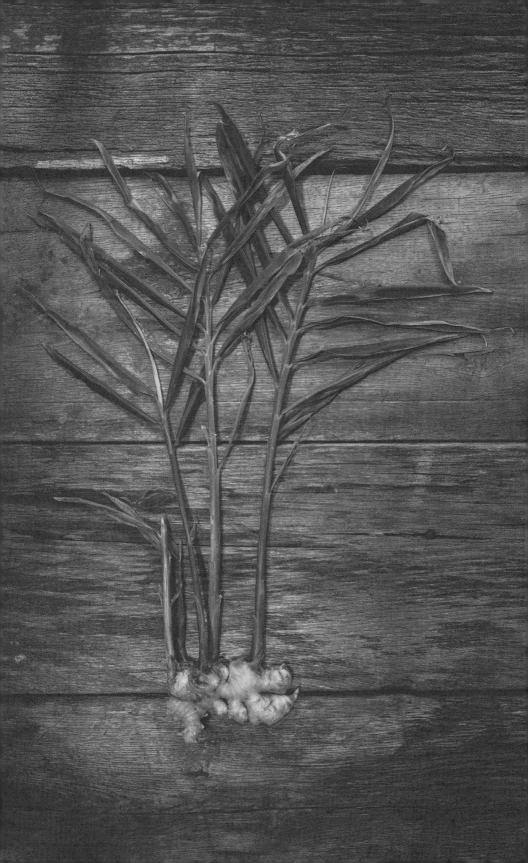

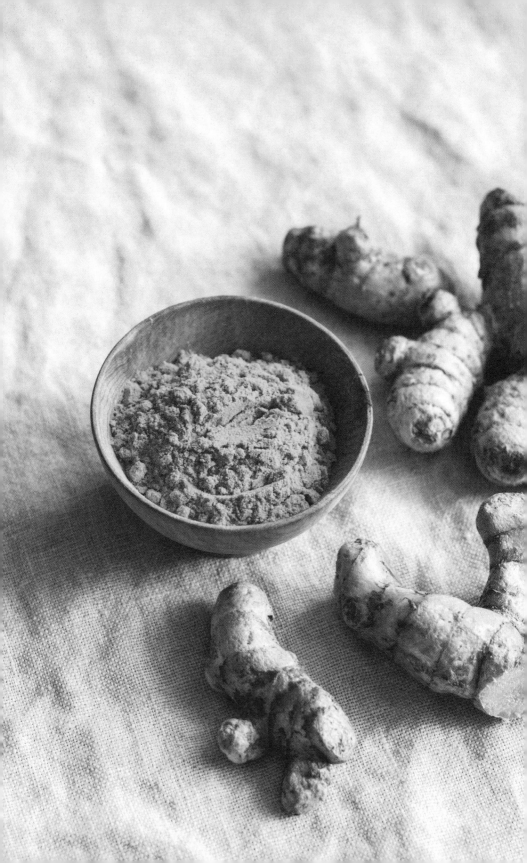

HOMEMADE FABRIC DYE ⓣ

By this point in your relationship with turmeric, it is not news to you that the stuff stains. If you use turmeric regularly, chances are you've had at least one *incident* wherein something in your house—a piece of clothing, a spot on the rug, a cutting board—is now permanently yellow. And not just kinda yellow. Yellow like a thousand burning suns. YELLOW. Well, guess what? You aren't the first to notice that turmeric is a powerful pigment. It's been used—along with fruits, vegetables, and flowers—to alter the color of fabric since ancient times. So, why not harness that staining power and make your own homemade natural fabric dye? It's easy, it's eco-friendly, and it costs almost nothing. Plus, the result is stunning. You can dye just about any fabric—clothing, table linens, bedsheets, throw rugs—just make sure you're using a natural fiber, such as cotton, wool, linen, muslin, or hemp. And remember that the longer you leave the fabric in the dye, the more vibrant the result. After that, this project is all about having fun! (And maybe making it look as though that apron you accidentally stained with last week's curry was meant to be yellow all along.)

Number of uses depends on the size of the item to be dyed

Continued

3 quarts water

½ cup salt

¼ cup ground turmeric

1. Combine 2 quarts of the water with the salt in a nonreactive pot and bring it to a boil, then add your fabric and let it simmer for 1 hour. This salt bath will help your fabric take the dye later on.

2. Remove the fabric from the salt bath. When cool enough to handle, wring it out and rinse the pot.

3. Combine the remaining quart of water and turmeric in the same pot, bring to a boil, then lower the heat and simmer for 15 minutes.

4. Remove the dye from the heat, add your fabric to the pot, and, using tongs or a large spoon, submerge the fabric. Allow it to soak for at least 5 to 10 minutes, or longer if you want to achieve more vibrant color.

5. When you're pleased with the color of your fabric, rinse it in the sink until the water runs clear, then hang it to dry (or dry it in a dryer). When your garment is in need of laundering, be sure to wash it with like colors for the first couple of go-rounds.

NATURAL AIR FRESHENER Ⓖ

There's no debating it: one of the best things about ginger is the way it smells. Fresh, pungent, kind of warm but also kind of lemony, its intoxicating perfume is like no other. To give your home a gingery scent, whip up this fresh and easy room spray. With nothing more than baking soda (a natural air freshener), ginger essential oil, and water, this stuff is the real deal— no gaggy fake smells, no overly perfumy lingering clouds, no weird chemicals. No headache! This recipe makes enough to fill an 8-ounce spray bottle. But, if you want to go bananas and stash a bottle in every room of the house, go for it! Just scale up all the ingredients. And feel free to add other scents you like. Lemongrass, mint, and citrus pair very nicely with ginger.

Makes about 1 cup freshener

1 tablespoon baking soda
5 to 6 drops ginger essential oil (and/or any other oils you like)
1½ to 2 cups water

1. Combine the baking soda and essential oil(s) in a small bowl. Stir well, then transfer the mixture to a spray bottle and fill with water. Shake well until the baking soda has dissolved.

2. Use the air freshener anywhere in your home or office. The spray is great in closets, bathrooms, and the kitchen!

NATURAL GARDEN PESTICIDE Ⓣ

Gardening—getting your hands dirty, connecting with the earth, living off the land—is a calming, centering, life-affirming pastime . . . until it *drives you completely mad*! I certainly love the *idea* of a garden, and when things go my way I'm giddy with excitement about the bounty it can pro-duce, but the insects, animal invaders, and other unwelcome guests make me insane. I thought casual, backyard gardening consisted of plunking a few seeds in the dirt, watering them every few days, and then literally enjoying the fruits of my (moderate) labor. But what are those brown spots on the big, once-beautiful leaves on my zucchini plant? And . . . what the?! Something ate *all* the lettuce last night? And heeeeeey! Where did those tiny holes in my tomatoes come from?! Come on! (By the way, praise be to the farmers, who endure *every*thing.) Fortunately, I have managed to find at least one way to wage war against garden pests without resorting to scary chem-icals. This spray, in which turmeric figures prominently, is full of all kinds of smells and tastes that bugs seem to dislike, and it can help turn things around in a garden that's suffering from common pests. Use it once a week, unless you have a full-on invasion of insects, in which case you can apply it more fre-quently. Once the garden starts to recover, use it every couple of weeks or so to get rid of those pesky buggers.

Makes about 12 cups spray

3 quarts water

2 garlic heads, cloves separated and peeled, roughly chopped

3 cups fresh mint, leaves and stems roughly chopped

2 tablespoons ground turmeric

2 tablespoons cayenne pepper

½ teaspoon liquid dish soap

1. Combine the water, garlic, mint, turmeric, and cayenne in a large pot and bring to a boil over medium-high heat. Lower the heat to medium and allow the mixture to simmer for 2 minutes. Remove from the heat and allow to steep overnight.

2. Strain the mixture into a large bottle or jug and add the liquid soap. Store it in a relatively cool, dark place. A garage or basement is perfect.

3. To use: Fill a spray bottle with the solution. Spray the mixture on the leaves of affected plants. Don't forget the undersides!

Note: Please make sure to use this spray with caution. It is a pesticide, after all, and can kill beneficial bees and bugs just as easily as it can wipe out the "bad" ones. Use common sense: Don't just spray this stuff broadly in your garden; target the plants and areas where you need some help and leave the rest alone. That way, you'll keep from harming the good guys.

DIY ACID-BASE INDICATOR ⓣ

One of the most valiant uses for turmeric (one that I have not, thankfully, had occasion to test) is as an antivenom for king cobra bites. Research backed and everything! Second on my list of favorite obscure uses for turmeric—only slightly less useful than the antivenom—is the fact that it can be used to make your own litmus paper. Litmus paper tests whether a substance is acidic or basic. Simply dip the paper into the substance you're testing, and it will change color depending on whether it is acidic or basic. Curcumin, the main compound responsible for turmeric's color, will turn red in solutions with a pH greater than 7.5. Pretty cool! But why exactly you would need to perform a litmus test at home? Well, in all likelihood you wouldn't need to, but science is dope, folks, and this experiment is fun and easy to set up with common household ingredients. After you make the strips, you can dazzle your friends and family by trying them out on all kinds of things from the fridge or pantry to see whether they're acidic or basic.

Makes 20 to 40 test strips

2 tablespoons isopropyl alcohol (rubbing alcohol)
1 teaspoon ground turmeric
1 or 2 coffee filters

1. Place the isopropyl alcohol and turmeric in a glass jar or other container with a tight-fitting lid. Stir or shake to

combine. Let the mixture sit, covered tightly, for at least 10 minutes and as long as several hours.

2. Meanwhile, cut your coffee filters into ½-by-2-inch strips.

3. Without stirring the turmeric that has settled at the bottom of the jar (you want to work with a clear, unclouded liquid), quickly dip your paper strips about halfway into the jar, then blot off any excess with a paper towel, or use a paintbrush to lightly paint the solution onto the strips.

4. Lay the paper strips on a nonporous surface to dry.

5. To use your litmus strips, pour a little bit of whatever liquid you want to test into a cup or jar, then dip in the strip and swirl it around for about 10 seconds. Take out the strip and observe the color!

Example of liquids to test:

- Vinegar
- ¼ teaspoon baking soda dissolved in ¼ cup water
- Lemon juice
- Milk
- Soapy water
- Tap water

Warning: *This is not food!* Rubbing alcohol is poisonous if ingested, so do not drink the turmeric extract. And, because isopropanol is flammable, do not work near an open flame.

GROWING GINGER AND TURMERIC INDOORS G T

I love growing stuff from food scraps. The windowsill above my kitchen sink is often crammed with an assortment of jars sprouting who-knows-what that I just couldn't possibly throw away. A handful of scallion nubs, an avocado pit, a pineapple top, the butt from a bunch of celery . . . But my favorite kitchen gardening project is regrowing ginger and turmeric from scraps. It couldn't be easier and results in not only more ginger and turmeric, but also an attractive houseplant!

Grows 1 plant

1 piece fresh ginger or turmeric
Potting soil
Water for misting

1. Soak the ginger or turmeric rhizome in warm water overnight to stimulate growth and rinse off any chemicals that might be present, including growth inhibitors which would stymie your whole project!

2. Fill a shallow, wide flowerpot with potting soil.

3. Place the rhizome with the eye bud (this looks a bit like the eye on a potato) pointing up and cover it with about an inch of soil. Mist lightly with water.

4. Place the pot in a spot that stays warm and gets filtered, not direct, sunlight.

5. Keep the soil moist, being careful not to overwater. A spray bottle works well.

6. After 2 to 3 weeks, shoots should begin to appear.

7. In a few months, when you're ready to harvest, pull up the whole plant, including the roots, remove a piece of the rhizome, then replant it and repeat the process.

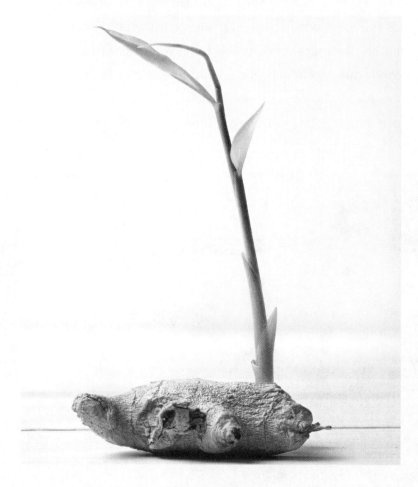

THE EASIEST WAY TO PEEL FRESH GINGER AND TURMERIC G T

Staring down a knobby, gnarly piece of ginger or turmeric, knowing that the only thing standing between you and a gorgeous recipe is that papery, brown peel covering every inch, nook, and cranny, can be enough to incite an adult-sized temper tantrum. Peeling ginger and turmeric is annoying! And as I've mentioned more than once, quite often I simply don't bother. But there are definitely times when texture and/or aesthetic does demand peeling, which is when I use the best tool I've got for the job: a spoon. Surprised? Well, it's true. The edge of a metal spoon works better than a vegetable peeler or even

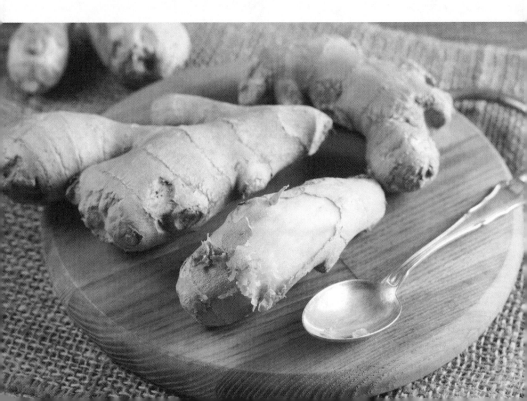

a sharp knife at getting around all the awkward curves and angles on a knob of ginger or turmeric. To do so, simply scrape the side of the spoon across the surface of the ginger. It'll get into all the bends and otherwise hard-to-reach places, easily removing the skin with such little effort you'll wonder what all your anticipatory crankiness was about in the first place!

TIPS FOR MAKING FRESH GINGER AND TURMERIC LAST LONGER G T

If you aren't juicing or otherwise going through large quantities of ginger or turmeric quickly, you could run the risk of ending up with a shriveled, dried-out piece of the rhizome (or a mushy, moldy one if your storage problems go another way) hiding out in your crisper bin. Such a bummer. You can, however, keep your ginger and turmeric safe from an untimely trip to the compost heap by relying on your freezer to keep it fresh longer. Here are three ways to go about it:

1. Freeze it whole. Just wrap it tightly in plastic wrap or store it in a freezer-safe container. When you need to use it, just take it out of the freezer and grate as much as you need, still frozen and everything!

2. Slice it. Lay slices of ginger and/or turmeric in a single layer on a baking sheet and freeze. Once frozen, store the slices in a resealable plastic bag or freezer-safe container. Then add them straight from the freezer to soups, tea, smoothies, or wherever you'd normally chuck in a slice of fresh ginger or turmeric.

3. Grate it. Press grated ginger or turmeric into an ice cube tray or blob it into little mounds on a baking sheet. Freeze it, then remove from the ice cube tray or baking sheet and store in a resealable plastic bag or freezer-safe container. You can then toss the frozen ginger or turmeric blobs directly into stir fries, soups, sauces, or smoothies. And for baking, all you have to do is pop the desired amount into a microwave and defrost it for a few seconds, then proceed with your recipe!

FIVE USES FOR LEFTOVER GINGER PEELS Ⓖ

If you cook with a lot of ginger, there's a good chance you're going to find yourself with a lot of ginger peels that might end up in the garbage can or, slightly better, the compost bin. True, they aren't the prettiest sight and they're not exactly a tender bite, but they're actually super flavorful and most definitely worth hanging on to. I like to stockpile leftover skins in a container in the freezer, adding to the stash each time I peel some ginger. Then, when I have a good, solid supply, I put those peels to use in one of these five ways:

1. Make a marinade for chicken or fish. For a spicy hit of fresh ginger flavor, combine a handful of ginger peels with 2 tablespoons of dark brown sugar, 2 tablespoons of soy sauce, 1 tablespoon of rice vinegar, and 1 teaspoon of sesame oil.

2. Make broth. Once you have a good-sized stash of peels, you can make this delicious, all-purpose broth to flavor all sorts of stuff from soups to smoothies to cocktails and more. Simply combine ½ to 1 cup of ginger peels with 4 to 6 cups of water in a medium saucepan. Bring the mixture to a boil, then lower the heat and simmer for 20 minutes. Remove from the heat and let steep for 1 hour. Strain and use immediately or store in the fridge for up to 1 week.

3. Make tea. Leftover peels work perfectly in tea, where they pack plenty of punch. Combine a tablespoon or two of leftover peels with a couple of slices of fresh lemon and 2 cups of water in a small saucepan. Bring the mixture to a boil, then lower the heat and simmer for 20 minutes. Strain the solids and sweeten, if desired.

4. Infuse vodka. This one is kind of a no-brainer and really couldn't be easier. Place a few tablespoons of ginger peels along with a thinly sliced lemon in a quart-sized mason jar. Add 2 cups of vodka (or rum or really just about any spirit you like). Cover the jar with a lid and let the mixture steep for at least 48 hours and up to 1 week, tasting it daily to see how you like it. Once the vodka is steeped to your satisfaction, strain out the solids and start enjoying your ginger-infused vodka.

5. Make a simmering potpourri. Fill your home with the clean, fresh scent of ginger and citrus with a stove-top simmer pot. Combine about ¼ cup of ginger peels with 2 sliced oranges, lemons, or limes and about 4 cups of water. Keep the mixture on a steady simmer over medium-low heat, adding water as needed throughout the day. Breathe deeply and enjoy!

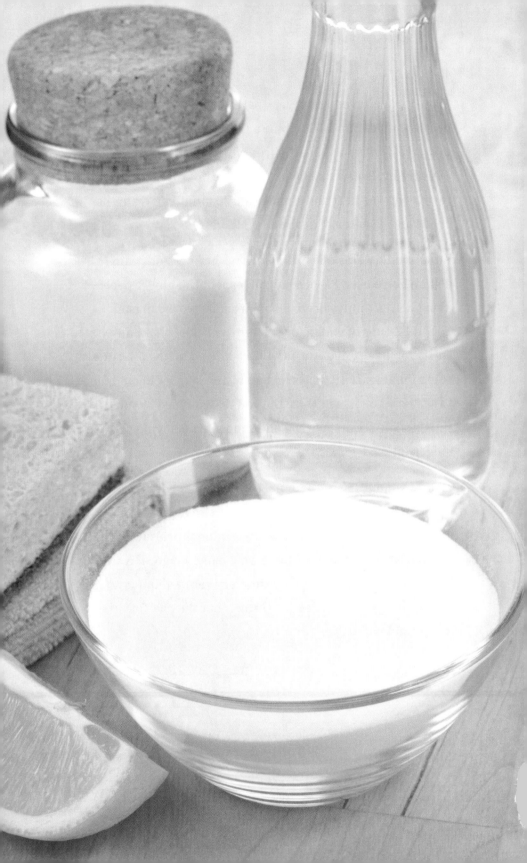

TIPS FOR REMOVING (SOME) TURMERIC STAINS Ⓣ

Your new favorite superfood has left its signature golden calling card on some of your old favorite dishware, linens, countertops, and, in all likelihood even your hands. Now what?! Don't fret—if you act fast and follow these stain-busting tips, you'll be able to salvage your stuff and your sanity.

PLASTIC AND CERAMIC DISHWARE:

1 cup hot water

½ cup bleach or white vinegar

Combine the water and bleach or vinegar in the stained dish or mug or in another container large enough to hold the item to be cleaned (mixing spoon, food processor parts, what have you). The solution can be scaled up, as necessary, for larger items. Soak the stained item overnight, then wash well with soapy water.

COUNTERTOPS:

1 tablespoon baking soda

1 tablespoon water or fresh lemon juice

Combine the baking soda and water or lemon juice to make a paste. Apply it to the countertop, then allow it to sit for 10 to 15 minutes. Scrub with a sponge, rag (perhaps from a T-shirt you've already stained with turmeric), or Magic Eraser until the stain is minimized and/or removed completely.

Continued

FABRIC (SUCH AS CLOTHING OR TABLE LINENS):

1 to 3 teaspoons baking soda or cornstarch

⅛ teaspoon liquid laundry detergent or liquid dish soap OR
   ¼ cup bleach

Bucketful of hot water

1. Here's where acting quickly counts the most! First, wipe off as much turmeric as you can, then sprinkle the baking soda or cornstarch onto the affected area. After 5 to 10 minutes, you should notice the powder soaking up some of the stain, which allows it to safely be brushed away.

2. Next, pour the liquid detergent onto the stain and scrub gently for several minutes on both sides of the fabric with a washcloth or soft toothbrush. Let the detergent sit for about 10 minutes, then wash your garment in a washing machine on its hottest setting. Dry in a dryer or in the sun. For some reason, sunlight has magical stain-lifting powers. Really!

3. And, of course, for stains on pure white fabric, there's always bleach. Add the bleach to the bucket of hot water and soak your white clothes or linens for about 15 minutes before sending them through the wash.

4. If all else fails, use the stained fabric for something else. Like, as a rag for cleaning your turmeric-stained counters!

ACKNOWLEDGMENTS

Many, many thanks to Ann Treistman, Aurora Bell, Isabel McCarthy, Nick Teodoro, and everyone at The Countryman Press who has helped nurture this project—you make me look so good! I have loved working with you.

To my agent, Sharon Bowers, the voice of reason and bottomless well of support—thanks for continuing to cultivate and support me as a writer. You've helped me find my voice and have taught me that being myself is the *only* way to actually get through writing a book. *Duh*, I know. You're the best. Truly.

Jamie Meadows—thank you for making me look good. Literally. It was a long time coming.

To my amazing friends and extended family, to whom I owe or have owed phone calls, emails, texts, and long-ago-borrowed Tupperware: thank you for your patience and support as I've finished this project. You're the best taste-testing, recipe-trying, cheerleading group of rock-solid supporters that ever there were. There's *no way* I would have been able to pull off a fourth (fourth!) book without you. Thank you all so much.

To my parents, who taught me that food and family and friends are inexorably intertwined, and that the table is the best place for good food, conversation, joy, and—more than anything—love. It is because of the two of you that I see the world though the nourishing, nurturing, creative, food-obsessed lens that I do. Thank you for believing in me, for raising me to be a little bit of a risk taker (and a little bit insane—but in a good way), and for teaching me to believe in myself. Thank you for the example you've set for me—in so many ways. I love you.

Mikey, as I was writing this book, concocting all sorts of wacky flavor combinations, I was often reminded of the tasting game we used to play when we were kids—you know the one I mean. While I can't quite *thank* you for the gag-errific chocolate-sauce-on-a-Dorito or the other assorted culinary "surprises" you fed me way back when (I, of course, would *never* have done anything of the sort to you, *wink wink*), I am grateful for the good-natured ribbing, the big laughs, the arguing, forgiving, love, and support that we have always shared. You're the best little brother in the world and I'm endlessly thankful that we are in this together.

Mitchell, my love, my best friend, and my partner in crime, you didn't just make this book possible—you make everything I endeavor to do possible. You are an enthusiastic taste-tester, a fantastic editor, an honest sounding board, and unwavering source of support. There is no greater gift. I am beyond thankful for your belief in me and also for maintaining your post as Chief Laundry Administrator, even in the face of turmeric stains. You are everything and I love you.

Sugar and spice and everything nice, that's what you, my little MJ and IA, are made of. I am so proud of who you are and who you're becoming. Kind, funny, smart, and sweet, you girls make it all worth doing. (Keep bringing the spice—that's the part that keeps life so exciting and fun!) I am one lucky mommy. I love you, my delicious little maniacs.

CREDITS

Page 13: © tenkende/iStockPhoto.com; page 14: © Naypong/iStockPhoto
.com; pages 16 and 63: © margouillatphotos/iStockPhoto.com; page 20:
© Quanthem/iStockPhoto.com; page 30: © enviromantic/iStockPhoto.com;
page 33: © NatashaBreen/iStockPhoto.com; page 35: © Mariha-kitchen/
iStockPhoto.com; pages 37, 103, and 149: © Foxys_forest_manufacture/
iStockPhoto.com; pages 39 and 40: © natashamam/iStockPhoto.com; page
43: © LauriPatterson/iStockPhoto.com; page 46: © Oksana_S/iStockPhoto
.com; page 55: © IgorDutina/iStockPhoto.com; page 56: © jirkaejc/
iStockPhoto.com; pages 60 and 113: © AnnaPustynnikova/iStockPhoto
.com; page 67: © Olha_Afanasieva/iStockPhoto.com; page 72: © luchezar/
iStockPhoto.com; pages 77 and 83: © ALLEKO/iStockPhoto.com; page
79: © SherSor/iStockPhoto.com; pages 86, 155, and 200: © OksanaKiian/
iStockPhoto.com; page 93: © joannatkaczuk/iStockPhoto.com; page 104:
© Mizina/iStockPhoto.com; page 109: © microgen/iStockPhoto.com; page
111: © Little_Desire/Shutterstock.com; page 115: © letty17/iStockPhoto
.com; page 116: © sveta_zarzamora/iStockPhoto.com; page 119: © undefined
undefined/iStockPhoto.com; page 123: © nerudol/iStockPhoto.com; page
124: © udra/iStockPhoto.com; page 133: © Piotr Krzeslak/iStockPhoto.com;
page 135: © SStajic/iStockPhoto.com; page 140: © CalypsoArt/iStockPhoto
.com; page 144: © yulka3ice/iStockPhoto.com; page 157: © GSPictures/
iStockPhoto.com; page 162: © Julia_Sudnitskaya/iStockPhoto.com; page
165: © MelanieMaya/iStockPhoto.com; page 167: © NikiLitov/iStockPhoto
.com; page 169: © YelenaYemchuk/iStockPhoto.com; pages 173 and 193:
© mirzamlk/iStockPhoto.com; page 175: © JuliaMikhaylova/iStockPhoto
.com; page 181: © eskaylim/iStockPhoto.com; page 183: © kazmulka/
iStockPhoto.com; page 185: © svehlik/iStockPhoto.com; page 187: © Makidotvn
/iStockPhoto.com; page 197: © Amy_Lv/iStockPhoto.com; page 199: © Beth
Hall/iStockPhoto.com; page 209: © Lubo Ivanko/iStockPhoto.com; page 210:
© Qwart/iStockPhoto.com; page 216: © Geo-grafika/iStockPhoto.com

INDEX